MANAGING
PHYSICAL
HANDICAPS

MANAGING PHYSICAL HANDICAPS

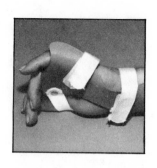

A
Practical Guide
for Parents,
Care Providers,
and Educators

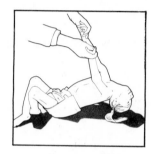

Beverly A. Fraser, R.P.T.
and
Robert N. Hensinger, M.D.

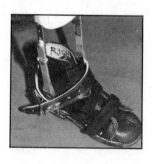

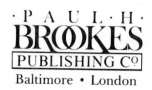

·P·A·U·L·H·
BROOKES
PUBLISHING CO.
Baltimore • London

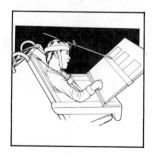

Paul H. Brookes Publishing Co.
Post Office Box 10624
Baltimore, MD 21204

Copyright 1983 by Paul H. Brookes Publishing Co., Inc.
All rights reserved.

Illustrations by Lewis L. Sadler, Medical Illustrator.

Typeset by Brushwood Graphics, Baltimore, Maryland.
Manufactured in the United States of America by
Universal Lithographers, Cockeysville, Maryland.

Library of Congress Cataloging in Publication Data

Fraser, Beverly A., 1938–
    Managing physical handicaps.

    Bibliography: p.
    Includes index.
    1. Physically handicapped—Rehabilitation.   2. Physical ther-
apy.   I. Hensinger, Robert N.   II. Title.   [DNLM: 1. Handi-
capped.   2. Rehabilitation.   3. Education, Special.   WB   320
F841m]
RD797.F72   1983   617   82-19716
ISBN 0-933716-30-3

Contents

Acknowledgments

The management approach to the care of physically handicapped persons described in this book has evolved over the past 9 years. Under the auspices of the Wayne County Intermediate School District in southeastern Michigan, we have worked cooperatively with classroom and administrative staffs to enhance the educational programs of severely impaired special education students. We thank the administrators of the following organizations: the Allen Park School District, which directly administered the program for much of this period; the Wayne County Intermediate School District, which encouraged development of the physical therapy/orthopaedic team clinic concept; and the University of Michigan Hospital, which permitted Dr. Hensinger to participate in our on-site school clinics. Together they provided a stimulating, flexible work environment and allowed us the latitude to develop our team approach. In particular, we thank Glenn Petersen, Walter Luke, Shirley Swegles, and Beatrice Gill for their support and encouragement.

This book centers around our recent work at Riley School, which provides special education programming for severely mentally and physically impaired students. We express our gratitude to the following Riley School staff members for their valuable assistance and personal time spent in reviewing the manuscript: speech-language pathologists Anne Baldwin and Patricia Cunningham; occupational therapists Ann Lehr and Melinda Mitchell-Reeber; physical therapist Jacqueline Bruno; nurse Karen Nycek; behavior analyst Tom Arkwright; teachers Elizabeth Fritz, Margaret Haver, William Holdsworth, Mary Mitrovich, and Jaroslaw Fylonenko; and instructional aides Joyce Comer, Jean Kreitzer, Kay Meszaros, and Vivian Stoychoff. Also, our appreciation goes to the total Riley School staff—custodians, instructional aides, teachers, support staff, and administrators—who helped us develop and refine our management program. We extend a very special thank you to the parents or guardians of the Riley School students whose photographs appear in this book. It is both their hope and ours that others will be helped by sharing in the experiences and accomplishments of the students of Riley School.

While most of Riley School's students live in private homes, some reside in nursing and group homes. We thank occupational therapists Sheri Staub and Mary Jo Kurily for working with us in coordinating in-home aspects of individual student management programs.

Any effective management program requires specialists who provide prescriptive equipment. We are privileged to work with Sandford Danzig, certified pedorthist, who designed the braces and customized shoes shown in Chapter 9; Pam Fillipus-Lupo, orthotist, who fitted the corsets in Chapter 7; and Edward Thomas, orthotist, and Bernard Herbert and David Barolo, orthotist assistants, who constructed the seating orthosis shown in Chapter 7. We are grateful to Barbara Schmitz, equipment consultant, for her advice, and to the equipment manufacturers and distributors who provided photographs of their products for this book.

One very special friend of Riley School, Bob McDermott, deserves special mention. On countless occasions, he has gathered community support from civic groups such as the Allen Park Kiwanis Club and private citizens to handle the pressing needs of individual students and enrich the school experience for all students.

Also, we thank the following persons for reviewing portions of the manuscript and contributing valuable suggestions: H. Sidney Heersma, M.D., Pediatrician; Thomas Greene, M.D., Orthopaedist; Genevieve Galka, OTR; and Shirley Swegles, Consultant, Michigan Department of Education. We acknowledge with gratitude the work of Susan B. Lillie, medical secretary to Dr. Hensinger, who supported our efforts.

Finally, we extend our appreciation to Melissa A. Behm, Managing Editor, and Roslyn Sassani, Production Editor, Paul H. Brookes Publishing Co., for guiding us during the development of this book.

Preface

Since 1974, we have provided a coordinated program of physical therapy and orthopaedic care to over 300 physically handicapped students—some for the entire 9-year period. All of the students have attended public school programs in southeastern Michigan supervised by Wayne County Intermediate School District, the third largest school district in the United States. Work with this student/patient population began at a time when physically and mentally impaired individuals were being sought out and placed in special education programs, in many cases for the first time.

We found that many of the individuals being placed in such programs had received only minimal medical, orthopaedic, and therapeutic care. They lacked proper adaptive wheelchairs and other positioning equipment. In fact, appropriate devices for use by individuals having severe physical impairments simply did not exist. Also, there was almost no mention of severely impaired persons in medical and therapeutic literature. It was apparent that severely impaired persons were essentially "forgotten" people.

There has been much progress since 1974. Attitudes among medical and teaching personnel and the general public have become more positive. Rehabilitation engineers, working with therapists, doctors, and special educators, have designed much specialized equipment to meet the unique physical needs of severely impaired persons. Manufacturers have begun to mass produce some of these items.

While what has been done to help physically handicapped persons is cause for encouragement, further progress remains necessary—progress that will require the efforts of all concerned. If this book helps parents, care providers, and educators in any way to deal more effectively with physically impaired persons, it will have served its purpose.

This book is dedicated to
Glenn Petersen,
Walter Luke, George Waters, and
the Riley School Staff.

Introduction

This book is intended as a practical guide for people who are involved on a day-to-day basis with children and young adults having serious physical handicaps. The focus is on the management of physical handicaps, particularly those experienced by physically impaired students attending special education school programs. The handicapped persons discussed in the pages that follow range in age from 3 years to the early 20s. All need some assistance from others—parents, care providers, educators, friends. Learning how to better manage the serious physical handicaps these individuals experience can help them enjoy more fulfilling, productive lives both as children and as adults.

DISTINGUISHING AMONG PHYSICALLY HANDICAPPED PERSONS

In writing this text, we found a need to differentiate among handicap severities because the severity of a handicap affects the extent of

1

assistance required from care providers. The terms used throughout the book to refer to physically handicapped persons are briefly described below.

Neuromuscularly Involved Individuals

Persons with physical handicaps who require a moderate degree of assistance from others often have handicaps that involve both nerves and muscles. We refer to such persons as "neuromuscularly involved"; that is, both nerve and muscle function have been impaired to some extent. Other individuals, who also require moderate care, experience muscle and bone diseases that do not involve the nervous system. When discussing these individuals, we mention the disease or condition specifically.

Severely Impaired Persons

In an educational context, "multihandicapped" is often used to refer to students who have both physical and cognitive problems whose combination causes such severe educational problems that they cannot be appropriately served in regular education programs or special education programs designed solely to meet needs associated with one of the impairments (Turnbull & Turnbull, 1979). In a fashion similar to educators' use of "multihandicapped," many health professionals have begun to use the term "severely multiply impaired" or simply "severely impaired" to refer to patients with *complex physical problems* (irrespective of the degree of mental impairment) that involve their total being. This terminology is used regardless of the specific medical diagnosis (e.g., cerebral palsy, encephalopathy). We use the term "severely impaired" in this sense throughout the book.

ABOUT THE BOOK

Managing Physical Handicaps is divided into four sections. Section I reminds us that individuals with physical handicaps must be regarded as "persons"—not as "patients"—who have many of the same needs as the rest of us. Chapter 1 presents a brief overview of society's treatment of handicapped persons in the United States. From the establishment of the institutions of the early 1800s through the current laws guaranteeing all handicapped children a free appropriate education, society's responses to the needs and problems of its handicapped members are examined. In Chapter 2, the reader is introduced to an emerging model of physical therapy/orthopaedic team management of handicapped persons that focuses on meeting the needs of the individual person. Physical therapy contributions to education are discussed in Chapter 3. Chapter 4 uses a question-and-answer format to address important questions about severely impaired persons. A number of the handicapping conditions and diseases frequently encountered in special education settings are discussed in Chapter 5.

After a basic description in Chapter 6 of normal body movement, including position and movement terminology and normal joint range of motion, Section II continues with a detailed look at many specific types of handicaps. The understanding of normal movement provided by Chapter 6 prepares the reader to learn about abnormal joint conditions that restrict normal motion in the spine, arms, and legs (Chapters 7, 8, and 9, respectively). Chapter 10 then discusses postural irregularities and abnormal balance reactions.

Chapters 11 through 13, which comprise Section III, address management of severely impaired persons specifically, focusing on their unique and extensive impairments and care requirements. Guidelines and tips concerning communicating, handling and positioning, and transporting severely impaired persons are discussed in detail.

Chapter 14, Section IV, looks to the future and suggests new directions in the treatment and management of persons with physical handicaps. Great strides have been made, but much more can be accomplished.

Appendix A contains a glossary of medical words and other terms that may be unfamiliar to the reader. These terms appear in bold type the first time they are used in the text. Appendix B contains names and addresses of equipment manufacturers/distributors of prescriptive equipment mentioned in the text. We recognize that more than one manufacturer may produce similar equipment. It is not the authors' intent to endorse any particular brand of equipment or recommend one piece of prescriptive equipment over another. Mentioned, however, are certain products that we have found helpful in providing a physical management program for the students with whom we have worked.

REFERENCES

Turnbull, H.R., & Turnbull, A.P. *Free appropriate public education: Law and implementation.* Denver: Love Publishing Company, 1979.

Section I

———

LOOKING BEYOND THE PATIENT TO THE PERSON

The Seriously Handicapped Population
Society's Response to Their Needs and Problems

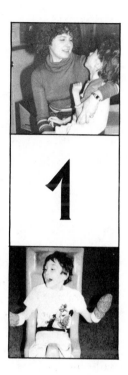

During a typical day, a physically and, perhaps, mentally handicapped student who attends a special education program is likely to come into contact with many different people. A parent or nursing home aide may help dress the student, apply prescriptive devices, and place him or her in a wheelchair. A driver will transport the student in a special vehicle to a school where he or she will most likely meet teachers, administrators, aides, custodians, therapists, nurses, behavioral experts, and other students. The student may participate in field trips to community parks, shopping centers, and entertainment events where he or she will come into contact with the general public as well.

All in all, the picture that can be painted today of interaction between handicapped and nonhandicapped individuals is a quite positive one. But, for the person afflicted with severe impairments, the situation has not always been like this.

HISTORY

Throughout its history, Western culture has been obsessed with physical perfection (Hallahan & Kauffman, 1978). It reacts both uncomfortably and negatively when faced with imperfection. Until as recently as the last decade, those unlucky enough to be severely physically and mentally impaired were often placed in institutions or sheltered in the protected environment of a private home. In either case, entire lives could be spent isolated from the stares, but also the stimuli, of the outside world.

When institutions for mentally and physically handicapped persons were first established in the mid-1800s, they were intended to be temporary boarding schools where mentally retarded and physically handicapped persons could go to learn skills that would allow them to be accepted in their communities. Unfortunately, lack of funds, insufficient concern for the rights of such persons, and popular philosophies of the day led to the abandonment of these institutions' original purposes. Conditions continued to deteriorate in the 1900s, and many institutions became dumping grounds for anyone the community considered "too different"—primarily society's mentally retarded members (MacMillan, 1977).

After World War II, conditions, especially for physically impaired persons, began to change. But change came very slowly at first. Gradually, improvements in wheelchair design, better bracing mechanisms, more effective artificial limbs, and the availability of special controls for motor vehicles began to make transportation more practical. Society learned greater tolerance as it became exposed to larger numbers of handicapped persons—in part, unfortunately, because of the great number of adults who returned from World War II, Korea, and Vietnam physically handicapped.

In recent decades, non-war-related factors have also contributed to increasing the number of physically impaired individuals in our society. Advances in medical science make it possible for handicapped children, who in earlier years would have succumbed during the newborn (**neonatal**) period, to survive beyond the critical infant years (Hallahan & Kaufman, 1978). New environmental risks, such as exposure to toxic and hazardous substances (**teratogenic agents**), have accompanied our evolution into a technologically advanced society. Social factors, including drug and alcohol abuse in expectant mothers and pregnancies in women under 20 and over 40, have also contributed to increasing the size of the physically impaired population (Seaver, 1967).

During the 1950s, helping the growing number of mentally retarded children became a special cause, spurred by a "parent movement" (Turnbull & Turnbull, 1979). Advocacy groups sprang up and brought their concerns to the attention of state and federal legislators. It was during this period that the Association for Retarded Citizens (ARC) was formed. ARC is a national parent-oriented group with state chapters dedicated to providing help to parents, individuals, organizations, and communities dealing with mental retardation. ARC's national headquarters is located at 2709 Avenue E, East, Arlington, TX 76001, phone 817-261-4961.

In the early 1960s, President Kennedy and Vice President Humphrey established the President's Committee on Mental Retardation as one response to the increasingly vocal concerns of such advocacy groups. The Committee's work helped to bring about improved opportunities for persons with handicaps, including the establishment of sheltered workshops, where some mentally retarded persons could learn productive work and earn at least a token wage (Turnbull & Turnbull, 1979). New Frontier programs initiated by President Kennedy were continued under the Johnson administration. Much progress was made duing the 1960s, increasing the public's awareness of the needs of physically handicapped and mentally retarded persons.

By the 1970s, the goals for handicapped persons that had begun with the advocacy movement of the 1950s were being more strongly articulated than ever before. Persons with handicaps were entitled to the same rights enjoyed by everyone else. Legislative and judicial acts began to ensure these rights. Closing down the sterile institutions (**deinstitutionalization**) and integrating impaired individuals as fully as practicable into everyday life (**normalization**) (MacMillan, 1977) became important principles for society to work toward. That these goals are becoming a reality is due in large part to the passage of two major legislative acts—Section 504 of the Rehabilitation Act of 1973, and Public Law 94-142, the Education for All Handicapped Children Act of 1975.

Section 504 of the Rehabilitation Act ensures that no otherwise qualified handicapped person shall be denied participation in or the benefits of, or be discriminated against in any federally financed activity or program solely by reason of his or her handicap (U.S. Department of Health, Education, and Welfare, 1978). Section 504 of the Rehabilitation Act of 1973 opened a new world of equal opportunity for handicapped Americans. Two years later, the key piece of legislation in calling attention to the concepts of de-institutionalization and normalization, Public Law 94-142 (Education of Handicapped Children ... , 1977), was passed by Congress.

PUBLIC LAW 94-142

PL 94-142 has three purposes: 1) to provide a free appropriate education for all handicapped children, 2) to protect the rights of handicapped children and their parents, and 3) to provide financial aid to the state and local educational agencies that administer special education programs (Surburg, 1981).

Providing a Free Appropriate Education in the Least Restrictive Environment

PL 94-142 entitles every school-age child to a free appropriate education regardless of the type or severity of his or her handicap. The key to ensuring a free appropriate education is the development of an individualized education program (IEP) by a committee of people closely associated with each student. In general, this committee, or IEP team, is drawn up during a meeting that includes the parents, school personnel, the student (when appropriate), and other individuals who will be providing consultative services. This committee is responsible for determining the eligibility of the student for special education services and for recommending an appropriate, individualized program for the student. The unique feature of the free appropriate public education (FAPE) guarantee is that each eligible student has an educational program based upon his or her own needs.

Typically, an IEP addresses physical, emotional, and educational needs. Both annual goals and short-term objectives are included, and an updated program is established each year. A student's success or shortcomings in meeting agreed upon objectives is measured continually. The program may be revised (by majority consent of all IEP team members) when necessary to reflect changes in the assessment of a student's performance. Every 3 years a complete reassessment of each student's functioning level and school placement is undertaken by a review team including at least an educational psychologist and a specialist in the area of disability along with appropriate support personnel.

Besides developing the IEP, one of the important issues that must be addressed in determining a free appropriate public education is that of the least restrictive environment (LRE), a concept sometimes referred to as **mainstreaming** in its implementation. PL 94-142 describes and sets the parameters for this principle by establishing alternatives to regular school placement. To the maximum extent possible, handicapped students are to be educated with non-handicapped students. Special classes and separate schooling are prescribed only when the nature or severity of the handicap is such that education in regular classes with the use of supplementary aids and services cannot be achieved satisfactorily.

Based upon these FAPE and LRE concepts, then, the school setting may differ for students with various degrees of handicaps. Many mildly impaired, higher functioning students can participate in regular education classes full time, aided by support services only as needed. In other cases, providing a free appropriate education in the least restrictive environment may mean placing handicapped students in a school with normal children while assigning them to a special education classroom for a part of each day. This placement provides the opportunity for handicapped students to participate in any or all regular education programs and activities. Alternatives can range from full-time placement in a regular education classroom to contact with nonhandicapped students in hallways between classes or on the playground. For many severely impaired children, a least restrictive environment may mean attending schools that are designed specifically to meet their unique needs.

In all programs, it should be stressed that programming for individual, eligible students must be flexible. Through constant monitoring of programs and re-evaluation of goals and objectives, students must be allowed to enter other programs as their needs change.

Regardless of their program placement, handicapped students require special kinds of help. **Physical therapists, occupational therapists, speech-language pathologists,** nurses, doctors, social workers, and psychologists must work with the school staff to help handicapped students benefit from the school experience. (Readers interested in learning more about IEPs may wish to consider *Special Education: An Advocate's Manual*. Requests for information about this 1981 manual should be directed to Michigan Protection and Advocacy Service for Developmentally Disabled Citizens, 230 North Washington Square, Suite 200, Lansing, Michigan 48933. The Michigan Department of Education also has a document that addresses this issue. *The IEPC Process—Team Approach Planning, Coordinating, and Implementing Services for Special Students* may be obtained by writing to the Michigan Department of Education, Special Education Services, P.O. Box 3008, Lansing, Michigan 48909.)

Protecting the Rights of Handicapped Children

The second purpose of PL 94-142 is to protect the rights of handicapped children (to age 21) and their parents. Due process hearings concerning the rights of handicapped children may be requested on the basis of four issues—education, identification, placement, and free appropriate education. If a disagreement should arise about any of the four issues, PL 94-142 provides procedures that should be followed as well as established timelines that should be observed. If disagreements are not resolved to the parties' mutual satisfaction, hearings may eventually be held at the local, regional, or state level.

**Financial Aid to State and Local Agencies
Through PL 94-142**

The third purpose of PL 94-142 is to aid state and local education agencies in providing for the education of handicapped students. Federal monies made available under the law are used to hire personnel to work in the school programs. Many occupational and physical therapists are funded in this manner. Funds also may be used to purchase special classroom supplies and equipment.

This part of the law has drawn attention to the lack of suitable equipment for positioning and transporting severely handicapped individuals that existed prior to 1975. Rehabilitation engineers and manufacturers, working with physical and occupational therapists and doctors, have responded by developing many new and very helpful products to aid with posture control and mobility. This is especially important with respect to severely impaired students, because better student positioning and mobility have shown themselves to virtually be prerequisites to achieving any degree of success in the educational process (Galka, Fraser, & Hensinger, 1980). For example, customized wheelchair seating systems (see Chapter 7) make it possible for bedbound handicapped persons to be transported to a school building. Also, the addition of head and body control devices (see Chapters 7 and 13) to standard and travel wheelchairs allows a student to focus attention on the teacher or a task without undesirable head and body movement.

It is this provision for financial aid in PL 94-142 that has been instrumental in creating support-staff teams to service severely impaired persons in educational settings. Indirectly, it has also led to evolution of the team management approach to physical therapy/ orthopaedic care that is discussed in Chapter 2.

PROFILE OF THE SERIOUSLY HANDICAPPED POPULATION

According to statistics provided by the U.S. Department of Education, 71,688 multihandicapped students between the ages of 3 and 21 were enrolled in special education programs during the 1980–1981 school year (P. Burns, personal communication, 1982). In Michigan alone, 2,202 students were identified as severely multiply impaired in the 1981–1982 school year according to statistics provided by the Michigan Department of Education (S. Swegles, personal communication, 1982). Included in this number is the student population discussed in Section III of this book.

As indicated in the Introduction, multihandicapped persons have both physical and **cognitive** problems which combined cause such severe educational problems that these students cannot be accommodated in special education programs created to address the needs associated with one of the impairments. This educational categorization of ''multihandicapped'' equates most closely with the medical classification of ''neuromuscularly impaired.'' Not included in the national figure of 71,688 multihandicapped students are the non-school-age multihandicapped persons in our society. It is apparent that a substantial number of seriously handicapped persons live among us.

One of the most common causes of severe impairment is damage to or deterioration of the **central nervous system,** which includes the brain and spinal cord (Hallahan & Kauffman, 1978). Brain damaged children are found to be equally distributed among races and social backgrounds. However, males with severe physical impairments considerably outnumber females (MacMillan, 1977).

Regardless of their chronological age, the ability of severely impaired persons to perform voluntary physical movement usually falls into the birth to 10-month **developmental age** range. In other words, a 10-year-old severely impaired boy may only have the motor ability of a 9-month-old infant. Some severely impaired persons have no control of their head, trunk, and limbs. Many obtain the ability to sit only in a supported position. A few learn to stand and walk with assistance. Even these activities, however, are accomplished in abnormal ways. Severely impaired persons may have dislocated joints and bony deformities, which often develop or become worse during the growth process. They are dependent upon others for their basic needs such as feeding, personal hygiene, and mobility.

PROBLEMS OF EDUCATING
SERIOUSLY HANDICAPPED PERSONS

To provide an appropriate school experience for severely impaired students, educators very quickly had to learn about and attend to the unique physical, medical, and intellectual needs of these special students.

Physical Problems

Providing safe transportation and modifying school buildings to accommodate severely impaired students was the first order of business. Many school districts purchased buses equipped with wheelchair lifts to bring students to and from school each day. Ramps were added to bring wheelchairs into the building and extra space was created to accommodate wheelchairs in classrooms, doorways and other passages, and bathrooms. Special bathroom fixtures had to be installed for students capable of using a modified toilet. Lavatories were required in each classroom for the convenience and protection of staff who changed diapers and were handling students with skin rashes or communicable diseases. Mats and other floor equipment were needed instead of desks and tables for students whose physical deformities required them to spend much of the day in a reclined position. Physical and occupational therapists helped to modify traditional classroom equipment for severely handicapped individuals and to train staff members in handling special students.

Medical Problems

Because of the extensive medical problems found among severely impaired persons, medication often must be given to students during school hours. Nurses were added to the school staff to monitor students' medical problems and supervise medications. Some students require specially prepared foods and individualized feeding methods. To meet their needs, it was necessary to prepare foods and provide individually tailored eating aids. Educators learned to expect the unexpected, to have lifesaving equipment at school, and to have medical emergency procedures well established. A good relationship with the local police/fire emergency service was essential.

Intellectual Problems

Many severely impaired students function at a very low mental level, or at least appear to do so. Instead of books, crayons, and paper, educators learned to provide toys and therapy equipment designed to stimulate the severely impaired child's basic senses of hearing, sight, smell, taste, and touch. Because many students' intellectual learning ability is limited, the educational programs often became centered around activities to increase movement and mobility. At the same time, efforts continued to determine impaired students' mental levels and to plan and carry out a meaningful educational program for each individual.

CONCLUSION

Special educators have made headway in providing educational programs for students with physical handicaps—especially severely impaired individuals. At the same time, it is generally recognized that much remains unknown about how to achieve the best educational results with severely impaired individuals. PL 94-142 wisely included parents and health specialists to work with special educators toward the goal of an education that truly meets each handicapped individual's unique needs. It is hoped that, by working together, this goal can eventually be reached.

REFERENCES

Education of Handicapped Children, Implementation of Part B of Education of the Handicapped Act. Federal Register, Vol. 42, No. 163. Washington, DC: U.S. Department of Health, Education and Welfare, Office of Education, 1977.

Galka, G., Fraser, B.A., & Hensinger, R.N.. *Gross motor management of severely multiply impaired students, Vol. II: Curriculum Model.* Baltimore: University Park Press, 1980.

Hallahan, D.F., & Kauffman, J.M. *Exceptional children: Introduction to special education.* Englewood Cliffs, NJ: Prentice-Hall, 1978.

MacMillan, D.L. *Mental retardation in school and society.* Boston: Little, Brown & Co. 1977.

Michigan Department of Education. *The IEPC process—Team approach, planning, coordinating, and implementing services for special students.* Lansing, MI: Michigan Department of Education, 1980.

Michigan Protection and Advocacy Service for Developmentally Disabled Citizens. *Special education: An advocate's manual.* Lansing, MI: Michigan Protection and Advocacy Service for Developmentally Disabled Citizens, 1981.

Seaver, J. *Cerebral palsy—More hope than ever.* Public Affairs Pamphlet No. 401, 381 Park Avenue, New York, NY, 1967.

Surburg, P.R. Implications of Public Law 94-142 for physical therapists. *Physical Therapy,* 1981, *61*(2), 210–212.

Turnbull, H.R., & Turnbull, A.P. *Free appropriate public education: Law and implementation.* Denver: Love Publishing Company, 1979.

U.S. Department of Health, Education, and Welfare. *Handicapped persons: Rights under federal law, §504 of the Rehabilitation Act of 1973.* Washington, DC: U.S. Department of Health, Education, and Welfare, 1978.

Physical Therapy/ Orthopaedic Team Management of Persons with Serious Physical Handicaps

An Emerging Model

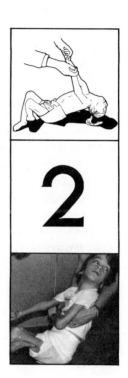

It is easy for medical professionals, when treating a patient, to focus on the particular ailment or handicapping condition that they are trying to correct. With such a disease-oriented approach, the needs of the patient as a total person may be overlooked. The "patient" may be exposed to seemingly endless periods of therapy, hospitalization, and bracing, as well as recurring surgery, while those treating him or her search for a technically perfect result. In the meantime, the "person" misses out on school, friends, and family—the broad spectrum of experiences that provide personal satisfaction and stimulate personality growth.

Some therapists and **orthopaedists** have begun to recognize that in the case of physical handicaps, a conflict can arise between treating the "patient" and caring for the "person." Recently, it has even been acknowledged that the disease-oriented approach to treatment of physical handicaps is often *unsuccessful* in overcoming these handicaps. Even more, such an approach may prove detrimental to

17

the impaired person and his or her family by creating false hope and the illusion that something positive is being done to improve the condition (Bleck, 1981).

To replace this limited disease-oriented approach, physical therapists and orthopaedists are turning to an analytical and function-oriented approach to patient care that emphasizes management of the handicapping condition—and, in the process, avoids prolonged, nonproductive treatment. In this chapter, we note past practices and explore current directions in physical therapy and orthopaedic care of persons with serious physical handicaps.

IMPROVED PROFESSIONAL AWARENESS

Public Law 94-142 has exposed increasing numbers of health professionals, among them doctors, dentists, and therapists, to the special problems of seriously handicapped individuals. Prior to 1975, many seriously handicapped children and young adults did not receive therapy (Fraser, Galka, & Hensinger, 1980). Physical, occupational, and speech therapists usually worked in a traditional hospital or clinic setting, but it was unlikely that seriously handicapped persons were brought to their attention. Furthermore, the low functioning level of severely handicapped individuals and the difficulty in transporting them often limited hospital visits to emergency care. Until 1975, most severely impaired individuals did not attend an educational program and, therefore, did not come into contact with the few therapists who worked with less seriously handicapped students in schools. It is often a school physical therapist who first identifies deformities and refers a student for orthopaedic care. As a result of severely impaired students' absence from classrooms, there were few referrals to medical specialists, such as orthopaedists, neurologists, and dentists. PL 94-142 brought many more physical therapists into school programs where they were confronted with chronic and complex handicaps experienced by severely impaired persons. In turn, their recommendations for medical and surgical evaluation contributed to greater involvement by others in the medical community.

THE PHYSICAL THERAPIST IN THE SCHOOL SETTING

A physical therapist, as defined by the U.S. Department of Labor, "plans and administers physical treatment programs for medically referred patients to restore function, relieve pain, and prevent disability following disease, injury, or loss of body part ... " (U.S. Department of Labor, 1977). Physical therapy was established as a profession in the United States long before this 1977 definition, however. In 1917, the U.S. Surgeon General's office instituted physical therapy for the purpose of physical reconstruction of war injured. Since that time, physical therapy has developed as a medically oriented profession currently serving 24 out of 27 medical specialities, e.g., orthopaedics, pediatrics, and neurology.

Traditionally, physical therapists have operated in a medical service environment that required direct patient treatment on a one-to-one basis. In the hospital setting, physical therapists treat patients of all ages with a variety of medical conditions. Treatment may consist of various modalities (e.g., ultrasound, infrared heat, **diathermy,** electrical stimulation, **hydrotherapy**), exercise, massage, manipulation, traction, and **ambulation** activities (e.g., training an amputee to use an artificial limb). Such treatment usually is provided in a well equipped physical therapy department. Treatment plans and progress reports are written in medical and therapeutic terms and care-related communication generally involves only the patient, the referring physician, and other health professionals.

In many hospital-serviced cases, physical therapy is successful in relieving pain and restoring function. Usually, only a short course of therapy is provided. Although the cost of such direct treatment is expensive, most patients, doctors, and physical therapists believe that the dramatic improvement that is brought about in the patient's condition is well worth the price.

In the school setting, physical therapists face a totally different situation. The passage of PL 94-142, the Education for All Handicapped Children Act, in 1975 (see Chapter 1), created a new dimension for physical therapists to work in an educational environment. This law mandated that physical therapy be available as a related service to assist a handicapped child in benefiting from special education, regardless of prospects for improvement in his or her physical disabilities. It went into effect at a time when the United States was experiencing an acute shortage of physical therapists. Furthermore, many of the modalities used by physical therapists in treating hospital patients were not appropriate for handicapped students whose needs focused on movement skills, positioning, and proper equipment. Some physical therapists considered the limitations placed upon their practice in education environments too confining, and returned to medical settings. As a result, school systems throughout the country experienced great difficulty in obtaining sufficient physical therapy support to meet their needs.

Those physical therapists who adapted to the school environment and began to work with severely impaired persons found that traditional therapeutic treatment rarely worked (Connolly & Anderson, 1978). Special techniques commonly used with less involved preschool children were difficult to perform because of the extensive deformities encountered and the fact that many students, because they were older, were heavy and awkward to handle (Bleck, 1979). Sometimes, therapists set unrealistic goals that were based on their experience with less involved individuals, only to become discouraged when small, nonfunctional gains resulted from treatment.

In school settings, physical therapists also found that emphasis was placed on the educational rather than the medical well-being of students (Levangie, 1980). Students were expected to be in their classrooms—not isolated from classmates in order to receive physical therapy in a "therapy room." This shift in treatment focus produced changes in physical therapists' thinking on service delivery methods, professional team participation, and record keeping. Physical therapists had to look for ways of incorporating therapeutic principles into students' daily activities. In order to do this, it became necessary to share knowledge of their specialty with others. Only by training parents, teachers, and instructional aides to assist in carrying out therapy plans, could cost-efficient, long-term service be provided to permanently handicapped persons.

The use of technical medical and therapeutic language, however, became an obstacle to effective communication in these efforts at team-delivered services. At best, the specialists' language was meaningful only in evaluation and progress reports directed to the referring physician. Therefore, school physical therapists were required to translate their medically written treatment plans into language easily understood by laypersons. Many therapists found this a difficult task. Maintenance of highly technical evaluation skills and a medical orientation is essential if a therapist is to serve as a school-medical liaison. While most physical therapists believe that hospital experience is a necessary prerequisite to a school-based position, adaptations to accommodate student and teacher needs in educational settings are necessary. As therapists are learning to communicate more simply, parents and teachers are becoming more familiar with aspects of medical technology, resulting in a continued narrowing of the communication gap.

THE ROLE OF THE ORTHOPAEDIST

An orthopaedist is a medical doctor who specializes in the preservation and restoration of the function of bones, joints, and muscles through surgery and other means (bracing). *Orthopaedist* is derived from the Greek words *ortho* meaning "straight" and "pais" meaning "child." Orthopaedists traditionally have treated persons of all ages. Recently, a subspeciality of orthopaedics has developed—pediatric orthopaedics. The practice of doctors who specialize in pediatric orthopaedics is limited to treatment of persons under 21 years of age, or those who are skeletally immature. These doctors are the specialists who most often treat the more severely impaired individuals, as well as persons with cerebral palsy and the other handicapping conditions mentioned in Chapter 5. At present, pediatric orthopaedists are usually connected with large universities or with teaching hospitals found in major U.S. cities.

Just as physical therapists found that they would have to adapt their approach when working with seriously handicapped students, orthopaedists discovered that severely involved persons often have multiple medical problems that complicate treatment. Many suffer from frequent seizure activity and respiratory infections that increase anesthetic risk during surgery. Severely impaired persons also have particular difficulty tolerating casts and braces and lack the ability to cooperate actively with a postoperative recuperative program.

However, the basic surgical procedures are similar to those used with less severely handicapped individuals and come under two major headings—**soft tissue surgery** and **bony surgery**. A soft tissue procedure involves lengthening muscles and tendons or releasing tight structures such as ligaments or capsules of joints. Bony surgery involves cutting bones to realign or fuse a joint in order to stabilize a part such as a foot.

Soft tissue surgical procedures generally require less time under anesthesia, a shorter period in a cast after surgery, and a faster return to normal activities than bony surgery. Soft tissue surgery may be considered to prevent a mild deformity from progressing to the point where bony surgery is needed. Its use is particularly appropriate with persons who have muscle imbalances that may lead to deformities of the hips, knees, and ankles. These imbalances are likely to produce progressive and severe deformities eventually interfering with the person's ability to sit or stand and leading to spinal deformities (see Chapters 7 and 9).

Orthopaedic surgery, particularly for the legs and feet, has proven successful in preventing pain and deformity and keeping impaired persons active. Orthopaedic surgery involving the arms and hands has been less successful for severely impaired persons. There are several reasons for this. First, severely impaired persons seldom have voluntary control over arm and hand muscles (i.e., they cannot move them on their own). Second, the sensations of touch and feeling are not normal, which serves to limit hand function. Third, it is difficult for surgeons to evaluate the benefits that might result from a specific hand surgical procedure when dealing with a severely impaired individual. Therefore, surgery on the arms and hands usually is approached cautiously. The surgeon should see the patient several times to assess functions of the hand under a variety of circumstances. It is imperative that the surgeon discuss each case at length with the attending occupational therapist and parent or care provider before deciding that such surgery is indicated for a severely impaired person (see Chapter 8).

Orthopaedists increasingly are recognizing the need to integrate the handicapped child into society, rather than segregrating him or her as a permanent patient (Bleck, 1979). As discussed in detail in other chapters of this book, orthopaedists are accomplishing this goal by reducing and, in some cases, eliminating bracing; shortening hospital stays; and timing necessary surgery to the convenience of the patient and the family.

EVOLUTION OF THE CONSULTATIVE APPROACH

As it became apparent that new systems of care would be needed, physical therapists and orthopaedists began to pool their knowledge of severely impaired persons and to work together in a team approach to patient management. For many, these considerations led to the evolution of a consultative rather than a medical service delivery system. Under such a consultative approach, the physical therapist and orthopaedist jointly establish the management program. The therapist is then directly responsible for input to the individualized education program, or IEP (see Chapter 1); demonstration of therapy techniques; and monitoring of progress achieved by each handicapped person. However, instead of the therapist providing direct treatment to the student each day, the practice of "hands on" therapy techniques is delegated to classroom staff and parents.

The actual therapeutic techniques are considered by many therapists and orthopaedists to be but one aspect—what might be called an "implementation" phase—of the physical therapist's role. Most techniques are comparatively easy to learn and may be performed correctly by classroom staff and parents after a short period of training. The therapist's principal expertise and value in the consultative approach to service delivery lies in evaluation and program planning (Bleck, 1979), that is, the development of a program of care and physical management individualized to the needs of the particular student.

In a school setting where there tend to be comparatively large numbers of students who require therapy, the consultative approach becomes almost mandatory. Relying on the more customary medical service delivery system, in which actual therapy is provided by a physical therapist, would be impractical from both resource availability and cost standpoints. Whereas a therapist in a consultative environment can handle a caseload of 75 or more students, a direct treatment–oriented program permits a maximum caseload of less than 30.

An added benefit of the consultative approach is that physical therapists who have learned to use it find that lines of communication are established with others concerned with the student (Sellers, 1980). Because educational goals for severely impaired students are physically oriented, it is necessary for everyone in the student's life to be trained in and use the same techniques in order for the student to learn optimally. Since physical therapists are new members of the educational team, they have much to learn from others who are veterans of the special education field. Shared experiences, it is hoped, will result in maximizing the effectiveness of student programming plans such as the IEP.

For most physical therapists, the use of the IEP's unfamiliar record-keeping system represents a major adjustment, since therapists must convert treatment plans into educational behavioral objectives that can be understood and, under the consultative approach to service delivery, often carried out by laypersons. It is important for parents and care providers to know that in public school, physical therapy goals must be included in the student's IEP (Levangie, 1980). This requirement helps to integrate physical therapy care into the process of managing the total "person." In addition, it provides a mechanism to ensure that each care provider in the total environment of the student understands all IEP goals and is better prepared to work toward them to the benefit of the student.

THE MANAGEMENT PROGRAM

The physical management program that has evolved from professional collaboration among physical therapists, orthopaedists, educators, and other specialists in the educational setting concentrates on correcting abnormal posture when possible, preventing further deformity to the degree practicable, and assisting the impaired person to adapt to the increased variety of his or her environment.

Experience of the past few years has shown that dramatic improvement in function is rarely possible among severely impaired students (Sommerfeld, Fraser, Hensinger, & Beresford, 1981). However, a management program that focuses on practical aspects of patient care can still be effective. The goals of such a program are as follows:

—to improve comfort and posture
—to maintain or improve joint flexibility
—to prevent or delay deformity
—to maintain surgical corrections
—to provide mobility through **gross motor** activities and selection of appropriate seating and transportation systems
—to help the patient adapt physically to varied environments

Achievement of these goals can make life a lot easier for the severely impaired person and for those who provide care to that person. For example, joint flexibility is needed so that care providers can dress and handle the person without strain. A parent, teacher, or care provider may need to use relaxation (see Chapter 10) and **range of motion** techniques (see Chapter 6) to separate a child's legs for a diaper change. Because much of the day may be spent on a mat or in special equipment, therapeutic positioning provides a foundation upon which to program other activities. Appropriate wheelchair selection and management is essential to meet the severely impaired person's home, school, social, and transportation needs.

The collaborative participation of those who work with seriously physically handicapped students on a daily basis is needed in order to carry out the objectives of this kind of a management program.

PHYSICAL THERAPIST/ORTHOPAEDIST RELATIONSHIPS

In the traditional relationship between physical therapist and orthopaedist, the therapist provided direct treatment to a patient as prescribed by the orthopaedist. Within the framework of the consultative approach, however, orthopaedists have challenged physical therapists to re-think many traditional treatment methods and focus their unique skills and training on a more productive type of service. With the encouragement of orthopaedists, physical therapists' responsibilities have grown beyond provision of direct treatment to encompass the roles of consultant, researcher, and orthopaedic assistant (Goldberg, 1975). In many instances, the physical therapist now is expected to supply information to the orthopaedist that aids in the diagnostic process.

Since the work schedules of most orthopaedists are demanding of their time, orthopaedists may call upon physical therapists to help explain to patients and their families combined orthopaedic and physical therapy management. While the surgeon should inform the patient and the patient's family about the risks, benefits, and technicalities of proposed surgery, the physical therapist may help answer questions about the management process. Some patients and their families find it helpful to talk to the attending physical therapist both before and after their discussion with the orthopaedist. The therapist can help the patient's family organize information they wish to learn from the doctor. This can be a great time saver for the surgeon and can help the family obtain the most important information during a medical/surgical conference. After the conference, the therapist may help with questions the family or handicapped person forgot to ask, or be able to contact the surgeon to obtain answers for them. However, therapists should not be asked to help the patient or parents decide whether or not to have surgery. This decision should remain strictly between the surgeon and the patient and family.

Following surgery, the attending therapist will monitor the patient's progress and keep the surgeon informed. With the amount of time spent in the hospital following surgery being reduced continually, school-age children are returning home and assuming their regular daily routines much sooner. The patient returns to the school program quickly. Therefore, school physical therapists are much more involved with postsurgical monitoring and the effect of surgery on the student's educational program.

CONCLUSION

We believe that a seriously handicapped person and his or her family should receive a truthful picture of the handicapping condition and management procedures, together with as accurate as possible a **prognosis.** It is only human nature for parents of handicapped children to want to hear about a miracle cure. They may travel considerable distances, going from doctor to doctor and therapist to therapist, to seek good news about their child. Pediatric orthopaedists and physical therapists spend a great deal of time attending continuing education courses and professional meetings, researching and reading, and contributing to professional journals in order to share ideas and to keep abreast of current treatment and management methods.

Promising treatments will not be kept a secret or withheld from scientific investigation. Parents can expect to find high quality orthopaedic and therapeutic care within their home state or nearby major city. Parents should, however, always feel free to ask their doctor or therapist about forms of treatment of which they have become aware. But, they should be prepared to accept the professional opinion that they receive in return. Doing so can save both anguish and expense.

Through the emerging model of physical therapy/orthopaedic team management for individuals with serious physical handicaps, treatment and care techniques are continuing to be improved and made more effective.

REFERENCES

Bleck, E. C.P. abroad: Winds of change. *American Academy for Cerebral Palsy and Developmental Medicine News,* 1981, *101,* 7–9.

Bleck, E. *Orthopaedic management of cerebral palsy. Saunders Monographs in Clinical Orthopaedics, Vol. 2.* Philadelphia: W.B. Saunders Co., 1979.

Connolly, B.H., & Anderson, R.M. The severely handicapped child in public schools. A new frontier for the physical therapist. *Physical Therapy,* 1978, *58,* 433–438.

Fraser, B.A., Galka, G., & Hensinger, R.N. *Gross motor management of severely multiply impaired students, Vol. I: Evaluation guide.* Baltimore: University Park Press, 1980.

Goldberg, K. The high risk infant. *Physical Therapy, 1975, 55,* 1092–1096.

Levangie, P. Public school physical therapist, role definition and educational needs. *Physical Therapy,* 1980, *60,* 744–779.

Sellers, J. Professional cooperation in public school physical therapy. *Physical Therapy,* 1980, *60,* 1159–1161.

Sommerfeld, D., Fraser, B.A., Hensinger, R.N., & Beresford, C.V. Evaluation of physical therapy service for severely impaired students with cerebral palsy. *Physical Therapy,* 1981, *61,* 338–344.

U.S. Department of Labor. *Dictionary of occupational titles.* Washington, D.C.: U.S. Department of Labor, 1977.

Physical Therapy Contributions to Education

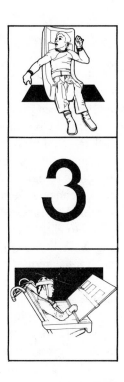

3

In spite of the fact that physical therapists have been required to work in public schools for only a few years, their work has already helped enhance the educational experience of handicapped students. Important contributions have occurred in the areas of evaluation, program planning, consultation, and research.

EVALUATION

Physical therapists are uniquely trained to evaluate **motor abilities** of physically handicapped and developmentally disabled persons. The use of the physical therapist's evaluation skills in screening for **scoliosis** and monitoring other deformities and posture abnormalities is described in detail in later chapters. Therefore, mention here of physical therapists' contributions to the evaluation process is limited to those concerning mildly handicapped students.

Two physical therapists have taken a first step toward developing a quick screening test that accurately detects a child with motor coordination problems (Kendrick & Hanten, 1980). Physical therapists Kendrick and Hanten investigated the possibility of differentiating 8-year-old learning disabled children from 8-year-old normal children by using motor tasks from the Devereux Test of Extremity Coordination. Their study showed that two coordination tasks—"thumb opposition," requiring the child to bring the tips of the thumb and index finger together, and "foot patting," requiring the child to pat the floor with the ball of the foot without raising the heel—can be accomplished by normal 8-year-olds but not by learning disabled children of the same age. These coordination tasks may be given to early elementary school children to identify potential learning disabilities. Quick screening tests are not diagnostic. However, such tests are useful in identifying children who should be examined for learning disabilities by physicians, educational diagnosticians, and teachers.

Another physical therapist has collaborated with a research specialist to develop a Basic Gross Motor Assessment test after analyzing research on minor **movement dysfunction.** This test is used to identify students in special education programs who require further physical therapy evaluation and, perhaps, a brief period of treatment followed by program planning (Hughes & Riley, 1981). The Basic Gross Motor Assessment includes nine tasks—standing balance on one leg with eyes open, standing balance on one leg with eyes closed, stride jump, tandem walking, hopping on one foot, skipping, target throwing with bean bags, yo-yo handling, and ball handling. It was validated and standardized and thus meets the requirements of a good assessment tool.

PROGRAM PLANNING

Evaluation often leads to program planning for the handicapped individual. Programs of physical activity and exercise are established, demonstrated, and monitored by the physical therapist, but carried out by teachers, care providers, and parents. Program planning in the form of a curriculum model for severely multiply impaired students was developed by the authors in association with occupational therapist Genevieve Galka (Galka, Fraser, & Hensinger, 1980). In later chapters of this book, program planning that involves a shared management approach to the care and education of severely impaired individuals is discussed. Such an approach is essential if a severely impaired person is to benefit from the least restrictive environment provision of PL 94-142.

Program planning may be just as important for mildly and moderately handicapped persons as it is for severely impaired persons if they are to enjoy normal socialization. Physical therapists have addressed this need by incorporating therapeutic techniques into such activities as dance (Wisecup, 1982), swimming, and other sports. The therapist designs the program to meet a specific individual's needs. Many times, the physical therapist works with a student's physical education teacher in developing such a program. This innovative approach allows the handicapped person to receive physical therapy in the form of pleasurable, socially oriented experiences, instead of having to undergo hours of boring exercise sessions isolated from friends and classmates. Of course, there are times (e.g., postsurgical care) when short periods of direct physical therapy will be needed. Any decision in this regard should be made jointly by the attending physical therapist and physician, and by the impaired individual and his or her parents.

CONSULTATION

Consultation involves sharing information both about the way in which others may help a particular handicapped person and about handicapping conditions. The consultative approach discussed in Chapter 2 is an example of the first type of consultation. Physical therapists have effectively used the latter type, general sharing of information, to increase nonhandicapped students' knowledge of handicapping conditions (Cecconi & Rothenburg, 1980) and to gain their acceptance of handicapped students in regular classrooms and schools (Westervelt & Turnbull, 1980).

RESEARCH

There has been an appalling lack of research concerning the effectiveness of physical therapy in treatment of certain handicapping conditions—especially **cerebral palsy** (Wolf, 1969). Concerned physical therapists are seeking to correct this situation by studying statistical and research techniques and conducting scientific studies—often in conjunction with physicians, educators, and research specialists. While the profession of physical therapy is based upon study of the physical, biological, and social sciences, methods of measuring the effectiveness of specific therapy techniques are needed. Research provides the answers—it gives the therapist an improved knowledge base that contributes to more effective patient treatment and management.

Research may be as simple as analyzing records of a handicapped person's condition or response to a treatment, or as elaborate as a study with similar subjects divided into groups receiving various types of treatments. An example of a recent record analysis study is work done by a physical therapist who examined the relationship of the **plantar grasp reflex** (see Chapter 9) to a developmentally disabled infant's future ability to learn to walk (Effgen, 1982). This study may help physical therapists and doctors predict the likelihood of a child's learning to walk independently—a valuable aid to realistic therapy program planning and to parent counseling.

Illustrative of more involved research using comparison groups is the work of the authors and several associates, who conducted a pilot study comparing the effectiveness of direct and supervised (or program planning) types of physical therapy service provided to cerebral palsied school students (Sommerfeld, Fraser, Hensinger, & Beresford, 1981). Results indicated no essential difference between the two methods in improvement of students' physical skills. This information may be useful to school administrators and therapists striving to provide high-quality yet cost-effective services.

In order for information obtained from research studies to be considered factual, it must be statistically significant after repeated testing. In both examples cited, the authors, in reporting their findings, stressed the need for continuing research. Replicated studies and broadened data bases help orthopaedists, physical therapists, and other researchers substantiate findings and contribute to improved care for physically handicapped individuals.

Unfortunately, laypersons often have misconceptions about such medical or therapeutic research. Without proper explanation and accurate information, they may imagine scenes of animal experimentation in isolated laboratories, or even episodes from old horror movies. In bygone days, research on handicapped children was perhaps not always carried out with parental consent or with the subjects' best interests considered (Jonsen, 1978). Today, however, all hospitals and treatment centers have an Institutional Review Board (IRB) that supervises all research projects (Batshaw & Perret, 1981). These boards, comprised of citizens from various walks of life, carefully monitor the work of research teams. Furthermore, parents or guardians of all persons who would be involved in a research project must give written consent before that person can be included.

Parents who are considering allowing their handicapped child to participate in a research project should ask about the study design and the credentials of the professionals who will conduct it. Parents and handicapped persons who participate can take pride in contributing much needed information to health and educational professionals, which, in time, will aide in improved levels of care.

Readers interested in learning more about the profession of physical therapy may contact The American Physical Therapy Association, 1111 N. Fairfax Street, Alexandria, Virginia 22314, phone 703-684-2782.

REFERENCES

Batshaw, M.L., & Perret, Y.M. *Children with handicaps: A medical primer.* Baltimore: Paul H. Brookes Publishing Co., 1981.

Cecconi, C., & Rothenburg, S. Model instructional program for mainstreaming handicapped children. *Physical Therapy,* 1980, *60, (8),* 1022–1025.

Effgen, S.K. Integration of the plantar grasp reflex as an indicator of ambulation potential in developmentally disabled infants. *Physical Therapy,* 1982, *62,* 433–435.

Galka, G., Fraser, B.A., & Hensinger, R.N. *Gross motor management of severely multiply impaired students, Vol. II: Curriculum model.* Baltimore: University Park Press, 1980.

Hughes, J., & Riley, A. Basic gross motor assessment. Tool for use with children having minor motor dysfunction. *Physical Therapy,* 1981, *61, (4),* 502–511.

Jonsen, A.R. Research involving children: Recommendations of the National Commission for the Protection of Human Subjects of Biomedical and Behavioral Research. *Pediatrics,* 1978, *62,* 131.

Kendrick, K., & Hanten, W. Differentiation of learning disabled children from normal children using four coordination tasks. *Physical Therapy,* 1980, *60,* 784–788.

Sommerfeld, D., Fraser, B.A., Hensinger, R.N., & Beresford, C.V. Evaluation of physical therapy service for severely impaired students with cerebral palsy. *Physical Therapy*, 1981, *61*, 338–344.

Westervelt, V., & Turnbull, A. Children's attitudes towards physically handicapped peers and intervention approaches for attitude change. *Physical Therapy*, 1980, *60*, 896–900.

Wisecup, R.C. Dance therapy. *Clinical Management in Physical Therapy*, 1982, *1*, (4), 26–27.

Wolf, J.M. The results of treatment in cerebral palsy. Springfield, IL: Charles C Thomas, 1969.

Questions and Answers about Severely Impaired Persons

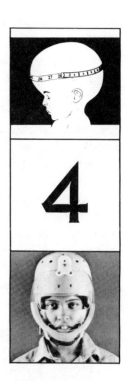

Most of us, at one time or another, find ourselves with many questions concerning severely impaired persons. We may not know where to go for answers or advice, or we may worry that certain areas are too sensitive to be discussed. This chapter uses a question-and-answer format to talk about topics that may seem troubling to those meeting severely impaired persons for the first time. Reference sources are listed for readers who would like more detailed explanations.

Are there certain physical characteristics that are typical of severely impaired persons?

Like the rest of us, severely impaired persons come in many shapes and sizes. However, most appear underdeveloped. For example, a 10-year-old boy might bear a physical resemblance to a "normal" child who is 4 years of age. A 21-year-old woman might be mistaken for a 12-year-old. Bodies of severely impaired persons are often affected by abnormal posture, irregular movement, and deformities of the back, arms, and legs. These conditions, which many times worsen with age, are discussed in detail in other chapters.

Are differences in head size another physical characteristic?

Yes. Head size of severely impaired persons may be too big **(macrocephalic)** (Figure 4.1), or too small **(microcephalic)** (Figure 4.2). Abnormal size of the head is determined by measuring the head's circumference at its greatest diameter and comparing it to the average for a person's age while taking into account body size and weight. In small heads, the size of the skull represents brain size and to some extent parallels brain function. Therefore, in most cases, microcephaly occurs because the brain has failed to grow due to damage or to a hereditary factor (familial microcephaly). In rare instances, the joints of the skull, called **cranial sutures,** are stuck together (fused).

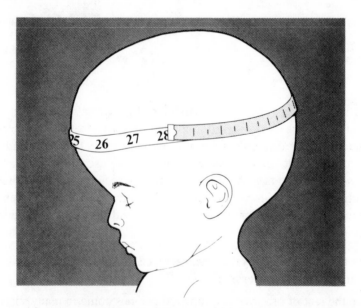

Figure 4.1. Hydrocephaly. This illustration depicts a 14-year-old girl who was born with an enlarged (macrocephalic) head. Note her prominent forehead. This head deformity was caused by the pressure of abnormal amounts of cerebrospinal fluid against the skull. She received a surgically implanted shunt to drain the extra cerebrospinal fluid early in childhood, and her head circumference has remained at about 28 inches since that time.

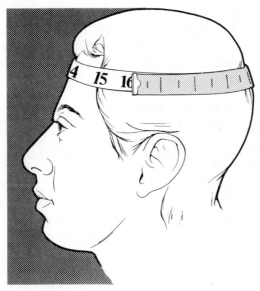

Figure 4.2. Microcephaly. The boy in this illustration also is 14 years old. He was born with an abnormally small (microcephalic) head. Compare his present head circumference (16 inches) with the girl in Figure 4.1 to see the contrast between hydrocephalic and microcephalic conditions. A normal young teenager has a head circumference of about 21 inches.

If this is the case, the brain is prevented from growing and surgery is required to allow the skull to expand and the brain to grow (Heersma, personal communication, 1982). Small head size may be present at birth and often accompanies mental retardation (Hallahan & Kauffman, 1978).

Macrocephalic head size is usually caused by **hydrocephalus**—an excess accumulation of **cerebrospinal fluid** within the brain. This condition is characterized by an enlargement of the head, including a prominent forehead. In all people, cerebrospinal fluid circulates constantly in the spinal column and inside and outside the brain to protect the central nervous system from sudden pressure changes and also to help supply nutrition to the system (Batshaw & Perret, 1981). In a person with hydrocephalus, circulation of the fluid is impaired or blocked by damage to the spinal column or brain. Excess fluid accumulates in the head and leads to wasting away, or **atrophy,** of brain tissue. Treatment consists of surgical placement of a tube (**shunt**) into the head, which is then connected to a second tube under the skin that runs to the abdominal cavity. This enables the blocked fluid to drain into the abdominal cavity. Hydrocephalus may be present at birth (**congenital**) or develop after birth (**acquired**) (Seaver, 1967).

What causes the physical problems found in severely impaired persons?

A safe generalization appears to be that brain and spinal cord damage—regardless of how it originates—is responsible for most of the extensive physical problems found in severely impaired persons. In the majority of cases, brain damage occurs before, during, or shortly after birth. (Specific causes are discussed in Chapter 5.)

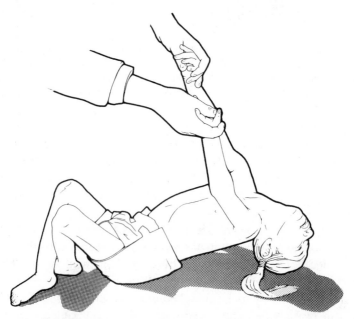

Figure 4.3. Head lag. A normal newborn will show a "head lag" much like the 4-year-old girl in this illustration. However, within the first few weeks of life, the normal infant will develop sufficient muscle tone to begin to control the head. *Caution:* Do not attempt to lift an impaired person by pulling on the hands or arms. We asked our artist to draw the child in this position to show an abnormal head lag clearly.

Occasionally, brain damage may occur long after birth. Usually this is the result of accidents, child abuse, or infections of the central nervous system (such as **meningitis**) (MacMillan, 1977). Complications following diseases (e.g., Reye's syndrome from a viral illness, encephalitis from measles) also may cause brain damage.

How does brain damage cause these physical problems?

The brain controls all bodily functions, including coordinated movement of the muscles. Severely impaired persons suffer brain damage that disturbs the balancing mechanism that controls the muscles, thereby upsetting normal muscle tension (**muscle tone**) (Seaver, 1967).

A brain damaged person may have too little muscle tone, called **hypotonia.** Among conditions in which hypotonia is found are a certain form of mental retardation known as **Down's syndrome** (formerly called mongolism) and a nonspecific, congenital condition that affects the nerves and muscles of infants. These children are referred to as **floppy infants** because they resemble "rag dolls" (Conner, Williamson, & Siepp, 1978). In both cases, low muscle tone causes loose joints, or **hypermobility,** and delays development. For example, an infant with low muscle tone will lack head control when pulled from a backlying position into a sitting position. This is referred to as **head lag** (Figure 4.3). A child with low muscle tone who is able to sit will do so with a rounded back and forward head (Figure 4.4). An older child with low muscle tone who is able to stand will do so with feet wide apart, legs turned out, hips bent, and back arched (Figure 4.5). In all three examples, the muscles are not able to adequately support the child against the pull of gravity.

Even an infant's tongue may be affected by low muscle tone. A floppy tongue can cause great difficulty with feeding. As a floppy infant matures, the muscle tone may change from too little to too much, or may fluctuate between the two extremes. In the case of Down's syndrome, muscle tone almost always remains hypotonic.

Brain damage may cause a child to have too much muscle tone, called **hypertonia,** which may lead to progressively more serious problems (Keats, 1970). A permanent increase in muscle tone causes stiffness in movement **(spasticity).** Eventually, permanent shortening of a muscle **(contracture)** may occur. Over time, the unbal-

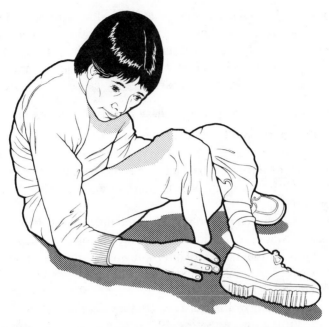

Figure 4.4. Low muscle tone seen in sitting position. The 10-year-old girl depicted in this illustration has learned to sit unsupported in a crossed leg, or "tailor," fashion. However, she cannot straighten her back or hold her head erect because of low muscle tone.

anced pull of muscles on bones and joints to which they are attached causes the bones to become misshapen and joints to dislocate, leading to **skeletal deformity.**

Are severely impaired persons deformed when they are born?

Most severely impaired persons have normal bone structure at birth (Fraser, Galka, & Hensinger, 1980). As noted previously, many deformities develop in response to brain damage and resulting muscle imbalance. For example, a set of muscles in the upper arm work together to allow normal **flexion** and **extension** of the forearm. As the muscle in the front of the arm (**biceps**) contracts, the opposite muscle at the back of the arm (**triceps**) relaxes to produce a smooth, controlled motion about the elbow joint. If brain damage causes the biceps to overpower the triceps, an elbow deformity may develop (see Figure 8.1).

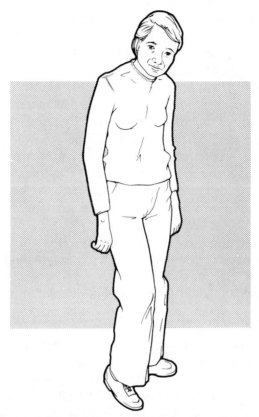

Figure 4.5.   Low muscle tone seen in standing position. This illustration of an impaired 16-year-old girl shows a typical standing posture for a person with low muscle tone—feet spread, legs turned out, hips bent, back rounded, and head forward.

Are deformities painful?

Most severely impaired persons are not in pain, although some pain may accompany hip dislocations, a frequently occurring condition (see Chapter 9). Severely impaired persons may become extremely uncomfortable, however, if they remain in one position too long (Galka, Fraser, & Hensinger, 1980). Just imagine how it would feel to sit absolutely still for an hour! If a normal person becomes uncomfortable while lying down, sitting, or standing, it is a simple matter to change positions. Since most severely impaired persons cannot do this, someone should change their position at least hourly during waking hours. Also, many of these persons cannot say that they are uncomfortable. They must be watched continually for signs of distress, such as flushing of the face, labored breathing, or increased bodily tension.

Hip and foot deformities may produce pain in teenage and adult severely impaired persons (Samilson, Tsov, Aamoth, & Green, 1972). Foot deformities may cause pain in persons who stand, walk, or wear shoes. A deformed foot will not fit correctly in a shoe. This can cause pressure on bony areas of the foot and irritation of the skin. Furthermore, a deformed foot has decreased surface for weight bearing, which may produce significant discomfort.

Although most severely impaired persons are capable of feeling pain, their response may be inappropriate. It is not unusual for a severely impaired person to laugh instead of cry when in pain. The possibility of inappropriate responses must be considered while watching such an individual for signs of discomfort or pain.

Can deformities be prevented?

In many instances, medical science doesn't know whether deformities can be prevented, or even kept from becoming more severe. Physical therapists use manual treatment to develop muscle balance and attempt to prevent or reverse early deformities in young children. Surgery such as muscle release or realignment may help prevent deformities or at least lessen their extent. But once deformities are well established—usually by age 7—emphasis shifts from prevention to therapeutic management. The goals of such a management program are to maintain the current functioning level, retard development of further deformity, and encourage the individual to develop skills within the confines of existing deformity (Bleck, 1979). Unfortunately, there is a scarcity of current research to prove the effectiveness of these methods (Sommerfeld, Fraser, Hensinger, & Beresford, 1981).

What are the physical abilities of severely impaired persons?

Most severely impaired persons function on a very low physical developmental level. Some have no control of their head or body and cannot even roll over. Many obtain the ability to sit only in a supported position. A majority of severely impaired persons are completely dependent on others for their basic needs, such as feeding, personal hygiene, and mobility.

What is the difference between severely impaired and cerebral palsied persons?

Severely impaired and cerebral palsied individuals differ principally in the severity of brain damage and resulting bodily disabilities. *Cerebral palsy* is a general term used to describe disabilities in movement and posture resulting from damage to motor areas of the brain or spinal cord before or during birth, or in infancy. Movement problems may involve various parts of the body. For example, muscle imbalance may occur in one, two, three, or all four limbs (Bleck, 1979). (Cerebral palsy is described in more detail in Chapter 5.) Cerebral palsied persons often become independent in activities of daily living. Many are conversant, hold jobs, and lead fairly normal lives.

Severely impaired persons have vast damage to the motor area of the brain. Usually, movement disorders are present in both arms and both legs **(quadriplegia).** Severely impaired persons may exhibit impairments in mental functioning. However, it is important to realize that not all severely physically impaired persons have deficits in their thinking (cognitive) abilities. Severely impaired individuals are much less likely to be capable of self-help or self-expression than cerebral palsied persons and are rarely able to attain the same degree of independent functioning in society that cerebral palsied and other handicapped persons can expect.

There may be considerable overlap of symptoms between cerebral palsied and severely impaired persons since severely impaired persons exhibit many of the problems encountered by cerebral palsied persons. In fact, severe cerebral palsied persons often are classified by educators as severely multiply impaired.

Do severely impaired persons have serious medical problems?

Severely impaired persons often suffer from a staggering array of medical conditions, ranging from chronic respiratory infections and cardiac problems to severe seizures and malnutrition. Physical inability to move normally or to clear mucus through coughing and nose blowing make severely impaired individuals highly susceptible to respiratory infections. Chest deformities that become increasingly severe with age serve to limit heart and lung function. Damage to the brain and nervous system is often demonstrated in the form of seizure activity. Medication needed to control seizures may alter muscle tone and responsiveness, creating additional movement problems for severely impaired individuals. Finally, the tremendous feeding problems experienced with many severely impaired persons make malnutrition a constant threat.

Why is feeding such a problem?

Eating and drinking probably are the most complex and frustrating problems confronting both severely impaired persons and those who care for them. The majority of severely impaired children experience difficulty with sucking, chewing, and swallowing. This presents a special problem to an abnormal infant who requires 10% to 25% more calories per day than a normal baby to maintain and gain weight (Conner, Williamson, & Siepp, 1978).

Both young and older severely impaired persons also often experience difficulty with the digestive process. Constipation tends to be a chronic problem for them because of lack of exercise and inadequate fluid intake. Some severely impaired persons experience gagging, vomiting, and swallowing of regurgitated food (**rumination**), which may be caused by behavioral or physical problems. Physical defects such as the **esophageal reflux,** which allows food to back up from the stomach **(Sandifer syndrome)** (Batshaw & Perret, 1981), also contribute to malnutrition. In addition, handicapped persons may have disorders of the small intestine that prohibit adequate absorption of nutrients.

Because of the extensive problems connected with feeding, it may be difficult for care providers to know if severely impaired persons are receiving sufficient food and fluid intake. Occupational therapists are specially trained to analyze feeding problems, prescribe feeding aids (Figure 4.6) and feeding seats (Figure 4.7), and design therapeutic programs to improve eating skills. In this way, they provide a life-sustaining service to severely impaired persons. The occupational therapist's expertise should be sought to teach care providers how to deal with eating and drinking problems.

It is beyond the scope of this book to discuss feeding problems in

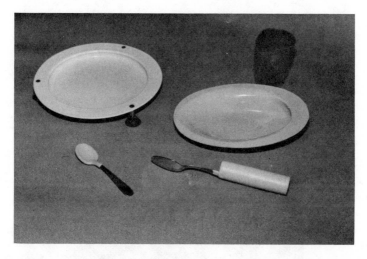

Figure 4.6. Feeding aids. The dish on the left is secured to a table by three suction cups in order to hold the plate steady for an impaired person. The one on the right is a scoop dish that is molded low in front and high in back to provide a surface that can help food land on a spoon. The spoon on the left is plastic coated to protect the teeth and lips. The one on the right has a rounded handle to make grasping easier. The cup in the background has a cutout for the nose so an impaired person can drink without tilting the head back. These are only a few of the specialized feeding aids available through Fred Sammons, Inc.

detail. However, there are many excellent texts on the subject. Listed below are a few of them for the benefit of readers who desire more information on feeding problems and skills.

> Campbell, P.H. *Problem-oriented approaches to feeding the handicapped child.* Ohio: Children's Hospital of Akron, 1976.
>
> Finnie, N.R. *Handling the young cerebral palsied child at home.* New York: E.P. Dutton & Co., 1975.
>
> Hanson, M.J. *Teaching your Down's syndrome infant: A guide for parents.* Eugene: University of Oregon, 1976.
>
> Sammons, F. *BEOK self help aids.* Box 32, Brookfield, Illinois 60513. 1980.

Do severely impaired persons require special foods?

Occupational therapists determine the type of food most appropriate for an impaired individual. The therapist may recommend baby,

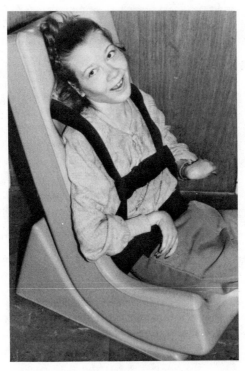

Figure 4.7. This student likes her adolescent-sized floor feeder chair. The chair may be positioned at various angles against the accompanying floor wedge. Floor feeder chairs are available in three sizes (small, medium, and large) from the J.A. Preston Corporation. They make excellent gift items for an impaired person or a special education program since they are easy to clean and may be used for therapeutic positioning as well as feeding.

mashed, chopped, or chunky food. Because the individual's diet must provide an appropriate nutritional balance, the therapist may work in conjunction with a nutritionist or pediatrician in developing a feeding program.

In cases where swallowing is difficult or impossible, **tube feeding** may be necessary. Generally, a nasogastric tube (inserted through a nostril into the stomach) is used, or in some cases, a special tube is inserted into a surgically constructed hole in the patient's abdomen (Batshaw & Perret, 1981). Food must be thin enough to flow through the tube. Such food is placed into the tube and administered either by gravity feed or with gentle pressure (Heersma, personal communication, 1982). In the school setting, the nurse supervises tube feedings after consultation with the attending pediatrician.

It is important to consult an occupational therapist or staff member familiar with a particular severely impaired individual before offering that person food. Offering the wrong food can even be life-threatening in certain situations. Well-intentioned volunteers may spend hours preparing special treats for a school or nursing home party, only to find that some of the children present cannot eat the food. To avoid disappointing the children, embarassing the volunteers, and possibly creating a health risk, this issue needs to be considered in party planning.

It pays also to be aware that severely impaired children sometimes eat unusual items! At the school with which the first author is associated, an occupational therapist casually placed her paycheck on a table in a classroom while feeding a child. Shortly after, she looked up to discover another student eagerly devouring the check!

Do severely impaired persons have control of bowel and bladder functions?

No, most do not have voluntary control of bowel and bladder functions (**incontinence**). Most severely impaired persons wear diapers and depend on others to change them and keep them clean. Disposable diapers are readily available for infants and young children. However, adults and persons who live in nursing homes may not use disposable diapers. Large, thick cloth diapers are often used instead.

There must be a sanitary method to care for diapers which are transported from home to school and back home. Care providers should keep an extra supply of diapers on hand at all times. Disposable gloves, deodorant spray, plastic bags, privacy screens, soap, and convenient accessibility to water should also be available. Because severely impaired individuals often do not achieve a level of physical activity sufficient to stimulate bowel movement, it is important to monitor bowel function for signs of bowel impaction (bloated abdomen and constipation). Similarly, bladder function should be monitored for signs of urinary tract infection (bloody or cloudy urine).

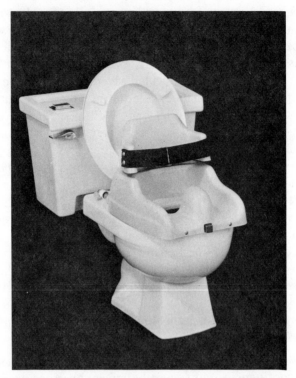

Figure 4.8. Child's trainer commode. This commode is designed to be mounted on a standard toilet. The back rest and foot rest are provided to support the child in a sitting position, and a belt is attached to the back rest for safety. The Child's Trainer Commode is available from Everest and Jennings. (Photograph courtesy of Everest and Jennings.)

Some severely impaired persons are able to indicate a need to go to the bathroom. In that case, without delay, they should be offered a urinal or helped onto the toilet or a special commode designed for handicapped persons (Figure 4.8). Assisting severely handicapped persons with toileting needs is an unpleasant, but necessary, job. Keeping the diaper (**perineal**) area clean prevents skin irritation and provides comfort and dignity to the handicapped person.

Is self-abusive behavior a problem among severely impaired persons?

Yes. Unfortunately, self-abuse does occur among severely impaired individuals. Typical kinds of self-abusive behavior included scratch-

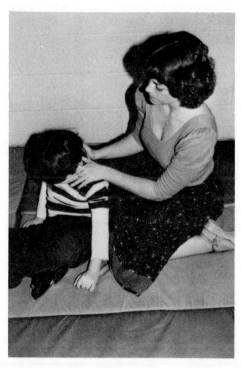

Figure 4.9. Elbow cuffs. The student in this photo, who has a history of chewing his hand, is wearing elbow cuffs to hold his elbows in a straight position and thereby prevent his hand from reaching his mouth. The cuffs were made by an occupational therapist. The student's teacher takes advantage of the situation and uses the straight arm position to help him learn sitting balance.

ing, hitting, biting oneself, and head banging. In such cases, it is necessary to protect the impaired person from him- or herself. A child may wear elbow cuffs (Figure 4.9) or hand mitts (Figure 4.10) to prevent injury to hands caused by biting (Figure 4.11) and to discourage hitting and scratching. Helmets (Figure 4.12) are often recommended as head protection for impaired persons who engage in head banging activities, as well as for those who experience seizures or are prone to falls.

Some schools employ a behavior specialist to teach the staff and parents how to eliminate or control undesirable student behavior **(behavior modification)**. Behavior modification may include techniques to increase or decrease the probability of a behavior occurring.

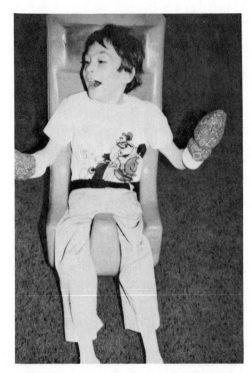

Figure 4.10. Hand mitts. This student wears hand mitts because abnormal reflexes cause him to bite his hand when it comes near his mouth. Usually he is a good sport about wearing the mitts to protect his hands from injury.

For example, it may be possible to increase purposeful hand activity by encouraging a student to hold a special toy. Since hand biting often results from reflex activity, it may be necessary to decrease this behavior by protecting the student's hands with mitts. These programs are planned and supervised closely by the behavior specialist, often in conjunction with a physical or occupational therapist. It is important to note that behavior modification programs are used *only* with the consent of the school staff and the student's parents or guardian (Martin, 1979).

Sometimes it is difficult for a visitor to a school for physically and mentally impaired students to know how to react to or cope with upsetting behavior displayed by students. The presence of a stranger may confuse or excite the students. It is wise for any visitor to remain

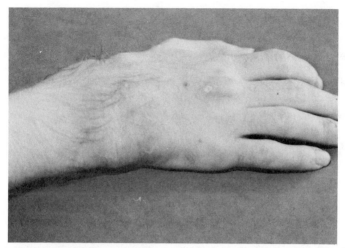

Figure 4.11. Hand injury caused by hand biting. Calluses on the knuckles were caused by constant hand biting. If this photo were in color, the entire hand would appear red and irritated.

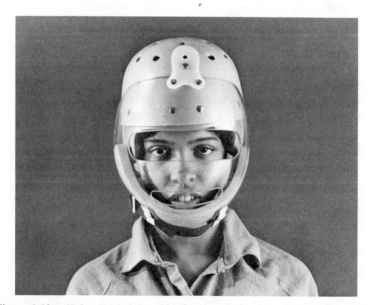

Figure 4.12. Helmet. A helmet with a face guard often is used by a student who is prone to falls. This helmet is available from Danmar Products, Inc. (Photograph courtesy of Danmar Products, Inc.)

with staff members and to follow their advice if confronted with a problem situation.

How can one communicate with a severely impaired person?

Because most severely impaired persons cannot speak, normal two-way conversation is often impossible. However, some impaired persons who cannot speak do understand what is said, and a number of mechanical aids have been developed to permit at least a basic level of communication. Beyond this, there are indirect methods (using physical, visual, and vocal prompts), relying on the impaired person's senses of touch, sight, and sound, to stimulate desired responses. Speech-language pathologists, who often are members of the support staff in a school program for severely impaired students, have proven to be most innovative in finding means of communication that work with particular individuals. This subject is discussed in greater detail in Chapter 11.

Are there professional organizations concerned with education and medical care of severely impaired persons?

Yes. At least three major professional organizations are concerned with the welfare of severely handicapped individuals (in addition to the Association for Retarded Citizens, which was referenced in Chapter 1). They are the Council for Exceptional Children (CEC), the American Academy for Cerebral Palsy and Developmental Medicine (AACPDM), and The Association for the Severely Handicapped (TASH).

The Council for Exceptional Children (CEC) was founded in 1922 for the purpose of advancement of educational programs for exceptional students. Its membership is organized into divisions for the physically handicapped, mentally retarded, learning disabled, communication disordered, behavior disordered and gifted. Of particular interest to readers dealing with severely impaired students will be the Division of the Physically Handicapped, which is concerned with crippled and health impaired children, including those home-bound and hospitalized. Educational professionals, para-professionals, parents, and others interested in the welfare of exceptional children are among CEC's members. Frequently, articles about severely impaired students appear in the CEC journal *Exceptional Children,* which is published 8 times a year, September through May. CEC headquarters is located at 1920 Association Drive, Reston, Virginia 22091. Phone: (703) 620-3666.

The American Academy of Cerebral Palsy and Developmental Medicine (AACPDM) was founded in 1948 to stimulate professional education, research, and interest in cerebral palsy and related disorders. At first, membership was limited to physicians. In recent years, other experienced health professionals, such as therapists and nurses, have been elected to membership. Also, the emphasis has broadened to include other developmental disorders. These changes reflect current trends away from individual medical and therapeutic treatment of the cerebral palsied patient and toward a multidisciplinary management approach to handicapped persons. The first AACPDM course on severely multiply impaired persons, which the authors were instrumental in presenting, was offered at the Academy's 35th annual meeting in 1981.

The AACPDM publishes a highly technical professional journal from England, *Developmental Medicine and Child Neurology.* While this may be of limited interest to lay-persons, the Association also provides free information about cerebral palsy and developmental disorders upon request. For further information, contact AACPDM, P.O. Box 11083, 2405 Westwood Avenue, Richmond, Virginia 23230. Phone: (804) 335-0147.

The Association for the Severely Handicapped (TASH) was founded in 1974 for those interested in providing educational opportunities for severely impaired persons. Members are advised of current problems, research findings, trends, and practices via a quarterly publication, *The Journal of The Association for the Severely Handicapped.* TASH's address is 7010 Roosevelt Way, N.E., Seattle, Washington 98115. Phone: (800) 336-3728.

By exploring the types of questions and answers included in this chapter, it is hoped that all of us will be more sensitive to problems likely to be encountered in educating and caring for severely impaired individuals. Later chapters amplify many of the points that have been raised here and should help to improve understanding of pivotal issues.

REFERENCES

Batshaw, M.L., & Perret, Y.M. *Children with handicaps: A medical primer.* Baltimore: Paul H. Brookes Publishing Co., 1981.

Bleck, E.E. *Orthopaedic management of cerebral palsy. Saunders Monographs in Clinical Orthopaedics,* Vol. 2. Philadelphia: W.B. Saunders Co. 1979

Conner, F.P., Williamson, G.G., & Siepp, J.M. *Program guide for infants & toddlers with neuromotor and other developmental disabilities.* New York: Teachers College Press, 1978.

Fraser, B.A., Galka, G., & Hensinger, R.N. *Gross motor management of severely multiply impaired students, Vol. I: Evaluation guide.* Baltimore: University Park Press, 1980.

Galka, G., Fraser, B.A., & Hensinger, R.N. *Gross motor management of severely multiply impaired students, Vol. II: Curriculum model.* Baltimore: University Park Press, 1980.

Hallahan, D.P., & Kauffman, J.M. *Exceptional children: Introduction to special education.* Englewood Cliffs, NJ: Prentice-Hall, 1978.

Keats, S. *Operative orthopaedics in cerebral palsy.* Springfield, IL: Charles C Thomas, 1970.

MacMillan, D.L. *Mental retardation in school and society.* Boston: Little, Brown & Co. 1977.

Martin, R. *Educating handicapped children: The legal mandate.* Champaign, IL: Research Press Co., 1979.

Samilson, R.L., Tsov, P., Aamoth, G., & Green, W.M. Dislocation and subluxation of the hip in cerebral palsy. Pathogenesis, natural history and management. *Journal of Bone and Joint Surgery,* 1972, *54*(A), 863–873.

Seaver, J. *Cerebral palsy—more hope than ever.* Public Affairs Pamphlet No. 401, The Public Affairs Committee, 381 Park Avenue, New York, NY, 10016, 1967.

Sommerfeld, D., Fraser, B.A., Hensinger, R.N., & Beresford, C.V. Evaluation of physical therapy service for severely mentally impaired students with cerebral palsy. *Physical Therapy,* 1981, *61*(3), 338–343.

Handicapping Diseases and Conditions

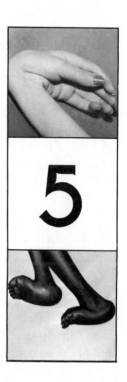

5

There are many different diseases and conditions that lead to physical handicaps. In this chapter, a number of those most likely to be encountered in a special education setting are discussed. While a detailed presentation is beyond the scope of this chapter—indeed the subject is so vast that complete coverage would fill many texts—we believe it is important for those associated with physically impaired populations to have at least a general understanding of these diseases and conditions. This will be helpful in:

—understanding how particular handicaps occur
—setting realistic individual objectives
—coping with sometimes inevitable loss of function
—learning special precautions associated with a specific disease or condition
—bridging the communication gap between parents, care providers, and medical professionals

Although a number of different diseases and conditions are discussed here, the effects on the body—the deformities that are produced—often are similar. These deformities are discussed independent of causation in Chapters 7, 8, and 9.

We'll start this chapter with diseases or conditions of the brain and spinal cord, known as **neurological conditions,** which account for most of the extensive physical impairments found among severely handicapped persons. Later, we shall turn our attention to diseases and conditions affecting muscles and bones, **musculoskeletal conditions.**

NEUROLOGICAL CONDITIONS

Under this heading, we discuss two neurological conditions commonly found among severely impaired persons (**encephalopathy** and cerebral palsy), accidents that produce injury (**trauma**) of the head, a congenital defect (**spina bifida**), and two diseases that affect children and adults (**poliomyelitis** and **multiple sclerosis**). A basic description of the anatomy and functioning of the central nervous system is not included; however, readers interested in this topic might consider *Children with Handicaps: A Medical Primer* (Batshaw & Perret, 1981).

Encephalopathy

Encephalopathy is a general diagnostic term used to describe any disease producing deterioration of the brain (**degenerative disease**). Encephalopathies may be caused by **metabolic diseases** (e.g., Tay-Sachs disease), diseases of the liver, diseases of the blood (e.g., sickle cell anemia, lead poisoning), and viral infections. An encephalopathy may occur either during pregnancy (**prenatal**) or after birth (**postnatal**). When working with a person having a diagnosis of encephalopathy, one must expect a progressive decrease in physical and mental functions leading ultimately to death. Periodic therapeutic evaluation of persons with encephalopathy is needed to note any change in their physical ability and to plan an appropriate management program.

Cerebral Palsy

Cerebral palsy is a general term used to describe disabilities in movement and posture resulting from damage to the brain or spinal cord before or during birth or infancy. Once the brain damage has occurred, it does not become progressively worse as with encephalopathies. However, the abnormal muscle tone and imbalance that are produced by the brain damage may become more fixed as the individual matures, leading to permanent deformities. It is estimated that cerebral palsy occurs in about 1.5 per 1,000 live births (Cruickshank, 1976).

Causes Numerous diseases or conditions may affect the immature brain and cause cerebral palsy. Prenatal causes include infection, ingestion of hazardous substances by the mother, chromosomal abnormalities, and abnormalities of the uterus and placenta. Conditions associated with the birth process include premature birth, lack of oxygen (**asphyxia**), and blood poisoning (**sepsis**). Postnatal causes include infection of the membranes covering the brain and spinal cord, called **meninges** (meningitis), and head trauma. Of those cases (about 60%) in which a specific cause of cerebral palsy can be identified, prenatal factors account for about 39%, **natal** factors for 56%, and postnatal factors for only 5%. In the remaining 40% of cerebral palsied patients, the cause is unknown (Batshaw & Perret, 1981).

Classifications There are two commonly used methods of classifying cerebral palsy conditions. One method considers the type of movement (motor) disability. Cerebral palsy may be classified as mixed if a combination of two or more of the below-mentioned types are present. Classifications are as follows:

Spasticity—refers to a permanent increase in muscle tone causing stiffness in movement. This occurs in about 50% of cerebral palsied individuals.

Athetosis—refers to involuntary, jerky movements. This condition is present in about 25% of persons with cerebral palsy.

Ataxia—refers to awkward movements and lack of coordination. About 25% of cerebral palsied persons are ataxic.

Rigidity—refers to continuous stiffness of muscles. Fortunately, this type of cerebral palsy is rare.

Tremor—refers to rhythmic, involuntary movement of certain muscle groups. It, too, is rare.

The other method describes the number of limbs having movement disorders (Denhoff, 1976). These classifications include:

Hemiplegia—involves the arm and leg on one side of the body (occurrence: about 40%).

Quadriplegia—involves all four limbs (occurrence: about 20%).

Triplegia—involves three limbs (occurrence: rare).

Diplegia—involves both arms and legs—legs to a greater extent (occurrence: about 20%).

Paraplegia—involves the legs only (occurrence: about 20%).

Monoplegia—involves one limb (occurrence: rare).

The two methods of classification may be used separately or in combination (e.g., spastic quadriplegia).

The movement disorders that are symptomatic of cerebral palsy may range from mild to severe. Many persons with mild symptoms require very little or no help from others. Persons showing severe symptoms—particularly the quadriplegia type—need a great deal of assistance from care providers.

Head Trauma

The two most common causes of head trauma in young children are automobile accidents and child abuse (MacMillan, 1977). The extent of trauma and resulting impairments varies greatly depending on the specific nature of the injury(ies). Like cerebral palsy, however, once the brain damage has occurred, it does not become progressively worse.

Both causes, to a large measure, are preventable. Use of proper child restraints considerably reduces the risk of head impact in the event of an automobile collision, or even a fast stop. Battered children suffer repeated severe injury that is inflicted intentionally by an older child or adults. Since child abuse usually takes place in private, it may be undetected until vast brain damage has occurred. Accurate statistics on child abuse as a cause of childhood trauma are not available. There is evidence, however, that infants and children who are especially irritable—particularly lower-than-average birth weight babies—are more likely to be abused than others (Park & Collmer, 1975; Sameroff & Chandler, 1975).

Spina Bifida

Spina bifida is a congenital defect of the bony spinal column characterized by incomplete closure of the spinal bones during fetal development. This defect may appear anywhere along the spinal column. Resulting damage may range from very slight to very serious.

Spina bifida occulta is a condition in which the spinal cord does not protrude through the opening in the spinal column. Persons with spina bifida occulta do not suffer neurological disability. In fact, the only outward sign of spina bifida occulta may be a clump of hair growing from the area involved—usually the low back.

Sometimes a tumor-like sac will protrude through the opening in the bone. This sac contains cerebrospinal fluid without nerve tissue. This is called a **meningocele.** Like spina bifida occulta, the meningocele form of spina bifida produces no sign of neurological disability. However, surgical correction is normally performed to reduce risk of meningitis and other complications.

If the sac contains the spinal cord or parts of it, it is referred to as a **myelomeningocele.** Paralysis is likely to be present below the site of the defect. Hydrocephalus (see Chapter 4) and meningitis are common complications. Surgery is capable of prolonging life, but is unlikely to be successful in reversing paralysis.

Poliomyelitis

Poliomyelitis, often called polio or infantile paralysis, is caused by a virus that attacks nerve tissue in the spinal cord or cranial nerves, or both. The damage caused by the polio virus can range from mild muscular weakness to complete paralysis and deformities. Fortunately, the Salk and Sabin antipolio vaccines were perfected in the mid-1950s, and the disease has subsequently been virtually eliminated in the United States. However, health statistics show a substantial drop in the percentage of American children vaccinated against the polio virus in recent years (World Health Statistic Report, 1976). Parents, in particular, need to remember that only through immunization can protection from poliomyelitis be assured.

Multiple Sclerosis

Multiple sclerosis is a slowly progressive disease of the central nervous system in which patches of scarring or hardening occur along the protective sheath of certain nerves. Symptoms may include muscle weakness; spasticity; and speech, hearing, and balance difficulties. The disease usually occurs in older adolescents and adults. Its course is characterized by **remissions** and relapses over a period of many years, with stress being a contributing factor to progression. The cause (**etiology**) of multiple sclerosis remains unknown.

MUSCULOSKELETAL CONDITIONS

People may have physical handicaps that result directly from defects or diseases of the muscles or bones, or both. These are known as musculoskeletal conditions. Even though such persons are not neurologically impaired, they may experience movement difficulties similar to persons who do suffer neurological impairment because of abnormalities in the muscles, bones, and joints of the arms, legs, or spine, or a combination of these.

Musculoskeletal conditions may be congenital or acquired, and their causes may involve genetic defects, infectious diseases, or accidents. Among the more common musculoskeletal conditions are **arthritis, osteogenesis imperfecta,** and **muscular dystrophy.** Scoliosis, another musculoskeletal condition, is discussed in detail in Chapter 7 and, therefore, not included here.

Arthritis

Arthritis is a condition in which pain and inflammation occur in and around joints. It often occurs in the elderly as a result of the aging process, sometimes referred to as wear and tear (osteoarthritis). However, arthritis may occur in people of all ages. Children may be affected with rheumatoid arthritis, a chronic and usually progressive disease of the joints that often leads to deformities. Unfortunately, both its cause and cure are unknown. Children with juvenile rheumatoid arthritis (sometimes called Still's disease) should be monitored by a physical therapist and treated during acute stages of the disease to postpone and, hopefully, avoid permanent joint stiffness and loss of motion.

Osteogenesis Imperfecta

Osteogenesis imperfecta is an inherited condition in which the bones are abnormally brittle and easily fractured. Sometimes, medical professionals are reluctant to share a patient's diagnosis with the patient's family, friends, and care providers. In the case of osteogenesis imperfecta, all those involved with the person *must* be aware of this diagnosis to prevent injury that may result from normal handling and contact. Persons suffering from osteogenesis imperfecta must be handled with extreme caution and moved as little as possible to avoid impact injuries. Never pull a person with osteogenesis imperfecta by the arms or legs and do not apply a strong touch—such as a grasp—to any part of the body.

Muscular Dystrophy

Muscular dystrophy is a general term used to describe a hereditary and progressive body weakness caused by degeneration of muscle fibers. There are two major types of muscular dystrophy: Duchenne and Landouzy-Dejerine.

Duchenne muscular dystrophy is only found in boys. Usually, muscle weakness is first noticed when the child learns to walk. Muscle weakness progresses until the boy is confined to a wheelchair—usually by early adolescence. Death generally occurs during early adulthood. Muscles of the person with Duchenne muscular dystrophy may appear overdeveloped, creating the impression of muscular strength. Actually, muscles are being replaced by fatty tissue, and muscle strength is decreased.

Landouzy-Dejerine muscular dystrophy has a later onset, usually in adolescence, and the progression of the disease is slower than in the Duchenne type. Weakness of the shoulders and arms is quite apparent and facial muscles are also affected.

It is important for parents and family members of a person with muscular dystrophy to receive genetic counseling. A genetic counselor presents factual information to family members regarding the origin, development, and cause of hereditary conditions. After considering this information, the family can make intelligent decisions about planning future children. Care providers also should be aware of the diagnosis in order to be prepared for deterioration of physical abilities and eventual death. Caution must be used in lifting a person with muscular dystrophy to avoid **dislocation,** particularly of the shoulders. Chapter 12 includes suggested lifting techniques that can be helpful in moving a person with muscular dystrophy.

Other Congenital Musculoskeletal Deformities

Infants may be born with deformities of the muscles and bones (congenital musculoskeletal deformities) for numerous reasons, frequently involving genetic and/or environmental factors. Such deformities commonly involve the spine, upper extremities, or lower extremities. These conditions are the same as many of the deformities described in Chapters 7, 8, and 9, respectively. Therefore, it is not necessary to present them here. The reader should be aware, however, that with early orthopaedic management most of these deformities can be either reduced in severity or corrected to a near normal condition by the time the child reaches school age (Hensinger & Jones, 1982).

CONCLUSION

The immature brain is more vulnerable than the mature brain to influences such as infections, malnutrition, chemicals and pesticides, metal poisoning, drug abuse, genetic conditions, and child abuse that can interfere with its normal health and function. This chapter has presented an overview of some of the more common causes of physical handicap. Once the disease or condition has become established, the prospects, generally, are quite discouraging. However, it is possible to prevent at least some of these abnormalities by proper prenatal medical care, immunization, good nutrition, and avoidance of hazardous substances.

REFERENCES

Batshaw, M.L., & Perret, Y.M. *Children with handicaps: A medical primer.* Baltimore: Paul H. Brookes Publishing Co., 1981.

Cruickshank, W.M. (ed.). *Cerebral palsy: A developmental disability.* Syracuse, NY: Syracuse University Press, 1976.

Denhoff, E. Medical aspects. In: W.M. Cruickshank (ed.), *Cerebral palsy: A developmental disability.* Syracuse, NY: Syracuse University Press, 1976.

Hensinger, R.N., & Jones, E.T. Developmental orthopaedics, I: The lower limb. *Developmental Medicine and Child Neurology,* 1982, *24*(1), 95-116.

Park, R.D., & Collmer, C.W. Child abuse: An interdisciplinary analysis. In: E.M. Hetherington (ed.), *Review of child development research,* Vol. 5. Chicago: University of Chicago Press, 1975.

MacMillan, D.L. *Mental retardation in school and society.* Boston: Little, Brown & Company, 1977.

Sameroff, A.J., & Chandler, M.J. Reproduction risk and the continuum of care-taking casualty. In: F.D. Horowitz (ed.), *Review of child development research,* Vol. 4. Chicago: University of Chicago Press, 1975.

World health statistic report, Vol. 29, No. 2. Geneva: World Health Organization, 1976.

Section II

ABOUT
PHYSICAL
HANDICAPS

Normal
Movement

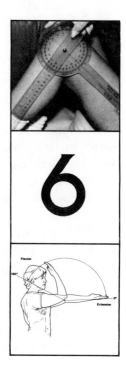

W e are more likely to appreciate the implications of physical abnormalities if we first have a basic understanding of normal movement. This chapter therefore begins with a brief review of terminology used by medical professionals to describe body positions and movements. A familiarity with these terms can help reduce the feelings of intimidation many people experience when discussing an impaired person's condition with a doctor, therapist, or nurse. Their explanations may seem like confusing medical jargon rather than helpful information if the terms used to describe the impairment are unknown to the person seeking advice. Also described in this chapter are the kinds and ranges of movement that occur around each major joint.

POSITION AND MOVEMENT

We'll start our review of terminology by looking at the body's position in space, then continue with directional terms applied to parts of the body, and finish with terms used to describe movement of the limbs.

Spatial Position

Most of the terms used to describe body position in space are ones with which we all are familiar—rolling, sitting, creeping, crawling, kneeling, and standing. Some of these actions can be performed in different positions, however, and the terminology used to describe the various body positions can become confusing. For instance, a person who is lying down can be said to be *supine* or *prone* or in a *sidelying* position. Understanding just what each of these terms means can be important in properly managing a physically impaired person. The three major kinds of lying position are defined below:

—When a person lies on his or her back, the position is called **supine.** Sometimes, the term *backlying* may be used to describe this position.

—When a person lies on the stomach or abdomen, the position is referred to as **prone,** or sometimes *facelying*.

—**Sidelying** describes a person lying on either the right or left side, usually with the legs slightly bent.

Directional Terminology

To identify sections or parts of the body in relation to one another, think of lines placed through the body at various angles. An imaginary line drawn from head to toes that separates the body into right and left halves establishes the **midline. Medial** is a term used to describe the body part closer to the midline. **Lateral**, the opposite of medial, is used to describe the body part further from the midline. For example, the mouth is medial to the ears, and the eyes are lateral to the nose. Similarly, **proximal** denotes something that is nearer to a point of reference, and **distal** something that is further away. Thus, the shoulder is proximal to the spine, while the hand is distal.

Now, suppose that our imaginary line were drawn in such a way that it divided the body into front and back halves. The front half is called **anterior** and the back half **posterior.** To illustrate, the nose is anterior to the face, and the ears are posterior to the nose.

Suppose that our imaginary line were drawn horizontally through the middle of the torso so as to divide the body into upper and lower halves. **Superior** pertains to the upper segment of the body, and **inferior** to the lower.

Movement Terminology

Bodily motion occurs at a union of two or more bones, called a *joint*. Much like directional terminology, movement terminology is described by opposing sets of actions. *Flexion* refers to a bending and *extension* to a straightening motion. Similarly, **abduction** is lateral movement, and **adduction** medial movement of the limbs. **Inward rotation** and **outward rotation** describe a turning from the shoulder or hip in which a limb rotates inward or outward, respectively. **Inversion** and **eversion** describe foot movement. Inversion occurs when the foot turns inward so that the sole is toward the midline of the body; and eversion describes a situation in which the foot turns outward away from the midline. **Supination** and **pronation** refer to motions of the forearm that turn the palm of the hand upward and downward, respectively. **Varus** indicates an abnormal curving of a part toward the midline, and **valgus** an angulation away from the midline.

These movements are possible because of three types of joint construction found in the limbs: hinge, pivot, and ball and socket. A *hinge joint* allows flexion and extension movement only. The knee is an example of this kind of joint. A *pivot joint* permits a rotary, or pivotal type of motion. This type of joint is located just below the elbow joint. A *ball and socket joint* allows several movements, including flexion and extension, abduction and adduction, and inward and external rotation. When these motions occur together, creating a circular motion of a limb, **circumduction** results. The shoulder and hip are examples of ball and socket joints.

Keeping movement terminology in mind, let's turn to a more detailed explanation of normal limb motion.

NORMAL JOINT RANGE OF MOTION

Normal joint movement occurs within a certain range that is measured by degrees within a circle or half-circle. The distance of the movement is referred to as *range of motion*. Therapists and doctors

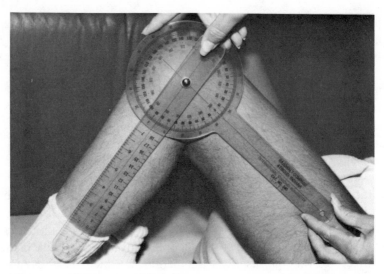

Figure 6.1. Goniometer measurement. In this photograph, a therapist is measuring knee flexion with a goniometer. As indicated on the goniometer, the knee is bent a little over 90 degrees.

use an instrument called a **goniometer,** which consists of two arms and either a 180-degree or a 360-degree scale, to measure the range of motion of **upper extremity** or **lower extremity** joint (Figure 6.1). For example, a typical reading for normal elbow motion is 0 degrees to 150 degrees. The 180-degree system of measurement used in this text is based on guidelines set by the American Academy of Orthopaedic Surgeons in 1965.

Learning how to use a goniometer is a normal part of training for therapists and doctors. The normal motion guidelines presented here do *not* prepare a reader to measure joints. Rather, the guidelines are presented to help provide an understanding of normal joint motion so that we can better recognize when substantial limitation occurs in joints that are deformed. The illustration of the human skeleton shown in Figure 6.2 can be used as a reference in locating the major bones that form joints of the spine and limbs.

Normal motion of the spine, the upper extremities, and the lower extremities are discussed below. Readers may find it helpful to perform the motions as they read about them.

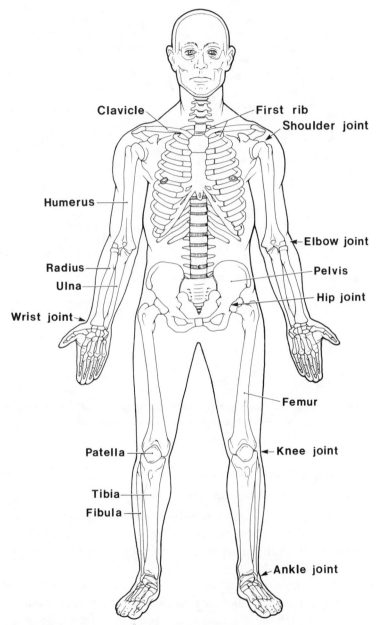

Figure 6.2. Skeleton. Shown here is an illustration of the skeletal structure of the human body. Major bones and joints are indicated.

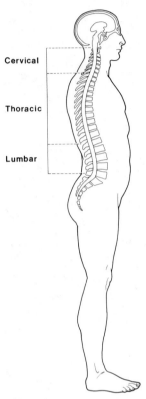

Cervical

Thoracic

Lumbar

Figure 6.3. Spine. This illustration of the human spine indicates the location of cervical, thoracic, and lumbar vertebrae. It also shows normal spinal curvature as viewed from the side.

Spinal Motion

The normal spine is composed of 33 vertebrae. The vertebrae work together to allow forward bending (flexion), backward bending (extension), sideways bending (lateral flexion), and rotation. Since flexibility varies greatly in normal persons, measurements of range of motion are not included here.

Abnormal conditions of the spine, discussed in Chapter 7, are measured by placing a goniometer on an X ray (**roentgenogram**) of the spine. Although the spine normally appears to be curved slightly forward and backward at different points when viewed from the side (Figure 6.3), it should look straight when observed from behind. In normal body alignment, the head should be directly over the pelvis. Spinal alignment may be demonstrated by running a finger along the tips of the spinal bones from the head down to the pelvis. Therapists often mark the skin over these bones with a skin pencil when screening teenagers for scoliosis (see Chapter 7).

Upper Extremity Motion

In order to coordinate the description of normal joint movement of the upper extremities with the discussion in Chapter 8 of the corresponding deformities of these joints, we'll start with the shoulder and progress to the fingers.

Shoulder The shoulder is a ball and socket joint that is capable of both single and combination movements—flexion, extension, abduction, adduction, rotation, and circumduction. The starting position used to measure joint mobility is with the arm resting against the side of the body, the elbow straight, and the palm of the hand touching the side of the leg. Shoulder flexion involves moving the arm forward and up. In a normal shoulder, it will be possible to raise the arm to a vertical position 180 degrees from the starting point. The return movement to the side is called extension. It should be possible with a normal shoulder to continue this movement beyond the starting point (backward extension) for about 60 degrees (Figure 6.4). From the same starting position, the arm may be lifted out away from the body and to a point above the head (abduction); or the arm may be moved across the body (adduction) to about 75 degrees (Figure 6.5).

Rotation may be demonstrated in either of two ways. The simplest is directly from the starting position by turning the arm in both directions—inward and outward—until the thumb points either toward or away from the leg. The method used by professionals for measurement purposes involves abducting the arm to 90 degrees, then flexing the elbow 90 degrees with the hand parallel to the floor (if standing), and moving the forearm up toward the head and down toward the hips while holding the upper arm stable. Total rotational range of a normal shoulder should be 180 degrees.

Elbow The elbow is a hinge joint that allows the arm to flex or extend. As indicated in Figure 6.6, normal flexion is approximately 150 degrees. Just below the elbow is a pivot joint that rotates the

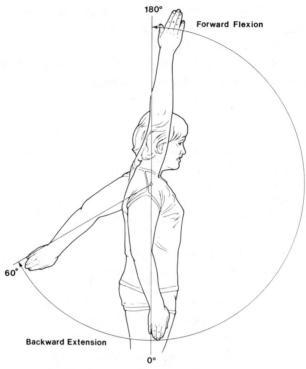

Figure 6.4. Normal joint range of motion for shoulder flexion and extension. From a starting point of 0 degrees, the arm can swing forward 180 degrees to a vertical position over the head and backward to 60 degrees.

forearm into a supinated or pronated position (Figure 6.7), with normal motion being 90 degrees in each direction.

Wrist The wrist is comprised of a number of small bones. Motions produced at the wrist include flexion and extension (Figure 6.8), and a sideways motion toward the radius bone **(radial deviation)** and toward the ulna bone **(ulnar deviation)** (Figure 6.9), as well as a combination movement (circumduction). As indicated in the illustrations, normal flexion approximates 80 degrees; extension, 70 degrees; radial deviation, 20 degrees; and ulnar deviation, 30 degrees.

Fingers and Thumb The fingers may flex, extend, abduct, or adduct. The thumb is capable of circumduction, allowing us to perform finely coordinated and highly skilled tasks **(fine motor**

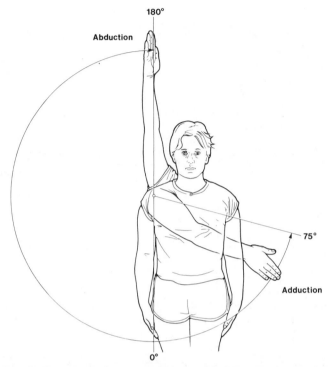

Figure 6.5. Normal joint range of motion for shoulder abduction and adduction. From a starting point of 0 degrees, the arm can swing (abduct) away from the body to a position of 180 degrees above the head and can move across the body to 75 degrees of adduction.

skills). Normal ranges of motion for the fingers are not included here because the focus of this book is on deformities of the larger joints that affect posture.

Lower Extremity Motion

The lower extremity joints are quite similar to those of the upper extremity in construction. We shall start with the hip and work downward to the toes.

Hip Like the shoulder, the hip is a ball and socket joint. It enables the leg to flex (Figure 6.10), extend (Figure 6.11), abduct and adduct (Figure 6.12), rotate, and circumduct. Normal range for the first four of these motions is indicated in the illustrations. Rotation is demonstrated by sitting on the edge of a table and

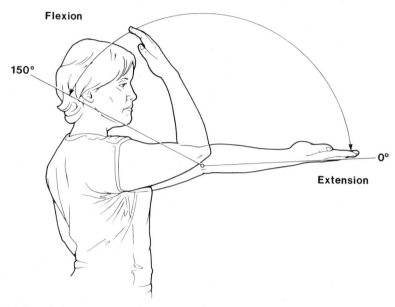

Figure 6.6. Elbow flexion and extension. Starting with the arm straight and the elbow fully extended, the forearm can move to a bent angle of about 150 degrees flexion.

swinging one lower leg laterally back and forth. Normal range is approximately 45 degrees in each direction.

Knee The knee, like the elbow, is a hinge joint. It moves in only two directions—flexion and extension, achieving a normal range of motion approximating 135 degrees (Figure 6.13).

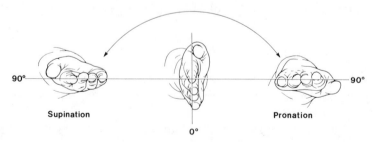

Figure 6.7. Forearm supination and pronation. Starting with the forearm in a neutral position indicated as 0 degrees, the forearm can rotate to turn the hand into a palm up position, reflecting 90 degrees of supination. Again starting from the neutral position, the forearm can rotate to turn the hand into a palm down position, reflecting 90 degrees of pronation.

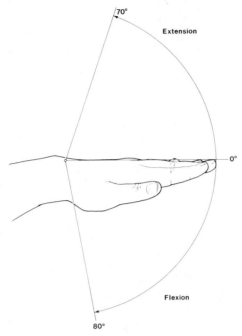

Figure 6.8. Wrist extension and flexion. Starting with the wrist in a neutral position of 0 degrees, the wrist can extend to raise the hand 70 degrees and can flex to bend the hand 80 degrees.

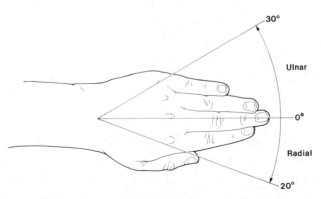

Figure 6.9. Wrist radial and ulnar deviation. Starting with the wrist in a neutral position of 0 degrees, radial deviation allows the hand to move 20 degrees sideways toward the thumb and 30 degrees sideways toward the little finger.

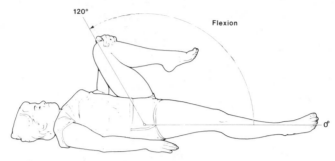

Figure 6.10. Normal range of motion for hip flexion. Starting from a neutral position of 0 degrees, the thigh can move to a 120 degree bent position.

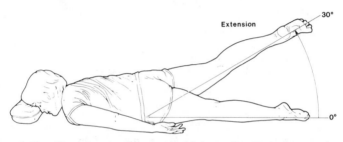

Figure 6.11. Normal range of motion for hip extension. From the neutral position of 0 degrees, the leg can move backward to an angle of 30 degrees.

Ankle The ankle is comprised of several small bones that enable the joint to move in flexion and extension (Figure 6.14), inversion and eversion (Figure 6.15), and circumduction. Normal ranges of motion are indicated in the illustrations.

Toes The toes flex and extend, and abduct and adduct. As with the fingers, detail is avoided here inasmuch as toe mobility has a limited impact on posture.

CONCLUSION

By understanding normal joint movement, we are better able to recognize deformities and appreciate their implications. Building upon the knowledge gained in this chapter, the next three chapters study abnormal joint conditions that restrict normal motion. Together, these chapters help prepare us to deal effectively with persons who have limited or abnormal joint mobility.

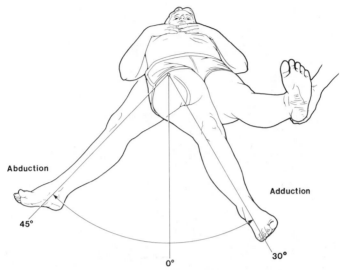

Figure 6.12. Normal joint range of motion for hip abduction and adduction. From a 0 degree neutral position, the leg can swing outward to an angle of 45 degrees and across the body to an angle of 30 degrees.

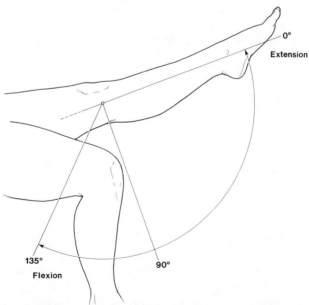

Figure 6.13. Normal joint range of motion for knee extension and flexion. Starting with the leg straight and the knee in full (0 degree) extension, the knee can bend the leg to a 135 degree flexed angle.

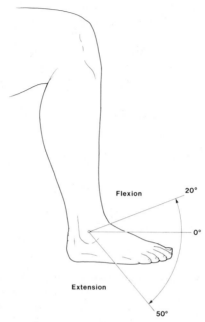

Figure 6.14. Normal joint range of motion for ankle extension and flexion. Starting with the foot in a neutral position, the ankle joint allows the foot to move upward into 20 degrees of flexion and downward into 50 degrees of extension.

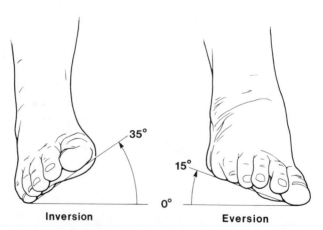

Figure 6.15. Normal joint range of motion for ankle inversion and eversion. From a neutral position of 0 degrees, the ankle joint allows the foot to turn inward to 35 degrees of inversion and outward to 15 degrees of eversion.

REFERENCES

American Academy of Orthopaedic Surgeons. *Joint motion method of measuring and recording*. American Academy of Orthopaedic Surgeons, 430 North Michigan Avenue, Chicago, Il, 60611. 1965.

Spinal
Deformities

7

Spinal deformities may occur in a sideways, forward, and/or backward direction—all three of the dimensions of normal spinal movement described in Chapter 6. Abnormal posturing of the spine is often called a *curve*. In this chapter we shall be concerned with three curves—scoliosis, **lordosis,** and **kyphosis**—that affect otherwise healthy, normal people, as well as neuromuscularly and severely impaired persons. In addition, a rare condition called *hyper-extension,* or **opisthotonos,** will be discussed.

Spinal curvatures may be either fixed (**structural**) or flexible (**functional**). Structural curves involve permanent changes in alignment of the spinal vertebrae. These changes cannot be corrected by simple positioning or manipulation. Functional curves may have an appearance similar to structural curves; however, permanent changes have not taken place in the joints and ligaments that connect spinal vertebrae. With a functional curve, spinal alignment may be improved by changing the person's position, through exercise, or by application of some type of force such as a corset, special seat, or scoliosis pads in a wheelchair. The more rigid structural curves require firmer measures such as braces to prevent progression of a curve.

Curves are named for the direction in which they produce an outwardly rounded appearance (**convexity**). For example, kyphosis is a backward curve that, in an abnormal (**pathological**) state, produces a protruding appearance to the back, often referred to as a hump. In addition, curves are identified by their location on the spine —neck (**cervical**), chest (**thoracic**), and lower back (**lumbar**) (see Figure 6.3). These terms may be used in combination to denote two areas of the spine, as in, for example, *thoracolumbar*. We shall begin our discussion of abnormal curves with scoliosis.

SCOLIOSIS

Readers may be familiar with the word *scoliosis,* a medical term meaning sideways curvature of the spine. In addition to a sideways bending, the scoliotic spine also has some rotation that causes a portion of the spine to turn toward the front of the body. As the spine rotates, it pulls the ribs along with it, thus creating a "rib hump."

Scoliosis occurs in about 2% of normal people, usually appearing during early adolescence when the spine is growing. Although boys and girls are affected equally, almost 7 times as many girls have progressive curves that require treatment (Scoliosis Research Society, 1981). The type of curve that occurs in otherwise normal adolescents is called *genetic **idiopathic** scoliosis* because it is inherited and its cause is unknown. The typical idiopathic scoliosis curve is S-shaped.

When scoliosis is found in children, teenagers, and adults with handicapping diseases or conditions, it usually develops as a result of muscle imbalance and assumes a C-shape. The C-shaped curve is a collapsing type of curve. Often, the pelvis is involved in the lower part of the curve and assumes a tilted position (**pelvic obliquity**). Thus, a neuromuscularly or severely impaired person with scoliosis sits in an unbalanced position, primarily resting on one buttock. Because of the oblique or tilted pelvis, the head of the **femur** on the side of the elevated portion of the pelvis is less well covered by the bony part of the pelvis (**acetabulum**) and, as a consequence, is subject to dislocation. This is a common occurrence in severely handicapped children, particularly those with spastic cerebral palsy. The pelvic obliquity and spinal curvature combine to make proper seating difficult.

Although X-ray measurement of a curve is standard for both S and C types of curves, detecting and treating curves in neuromuscularly and severely impaired individuals require unique approaches quite different from those used with otherwise normal teenagers. It is for this reason that further discussion of scoliosis is presented in two parts—one dealing with otherwise normal adolescents, and the second concentrating on persons who are neuromuscularly and severely involved.

Scoliosis in the Otherwise Normal Adolescent

Scoliosis may be discovered by parents who notice a child's poor posture, by a physical therapist, nurse, or physical education teacher during a school screening program, or by a family doctor during a routine physical exam. In early stages it is painless, but occasionally it may be brought to a doctor's attention by a teenager complaining of back pain. Parents and teenagers should be alert to the following telltale signs of scoliosis:

—one shoulder appearing higher than the other
—one shoulder blade (**scapula**) being more prominent than the other
—one side of the waist showing a more prominent indentation than the other
—one hip appearing higher than the other

Anyone suspected of having scoliosis should be promptly referred to an orthopaedist.

Scoliosis Identification and Measurement Early identification of scoliosis is important since mild cases, either functional or structural, respond best to orthopaedic treatment (Cailliet, 1975). Usually, scoliosis is first detected by a visual examination that includes the forward bending test. In order to perform this simple test, the examiner stands directly behind the person, who bends forward at the waist with the arms hanging freely in an extended position. In this position, the person's vertebral projections (**spinous**

processes) are more visible and smaller curves can be detected more easily. The forward bending position also accentuates the rib hump in the thoracic and lumbar areas of the spine.

Once scoliosis is detected, X rays are obtained to document the state of the curve—the degree of curvature and its pattern. X rays are evaluated using the Cobb method, which is the international procedure for measuring curves. Using this method, a mild curve measures approximately 20–40 degrees, a moderate curve 40–60 degrees, and a severe curve 60 degrees and above. When taking the X ray, it is important that the patient be placed in a position that can be replicated on later testing occasions. This way, films taken over several years can document progress accurately. The standing position is preferred during the X ray. The spine tends to stretch out when a person is reclining so that a less accurate picture of the curve is obtained in this position. Since many neuromuscularly and severely impaired persons are unable to stand, X rays of the spine may have to be taken in a sitting or, as a last resort, a recumbent (reclining) position.

Treatment   Nonsurgical treatment of scoliosis in the otherwise normal adolescent includes bracing to prevent progression of a mild curve. Recently, a device that provides intermittent or electrical stimulation at night has been used in the management of idiopathic scoliosis as a substitute for bracing. While still experimental, this device shows great promise. Traction and casts are used primarily for treatment of severe curves prior to surgery, where their use has been shown to improve the surgical correction by making a rigid spine more flexible. A cast or brace is used subsequent to surgery to support the trunk during healing.

Only surgical treatment corrects a curve. A common surgical procedure involves *spinal fusion*. In this procedure, the outer portion of involved vertebrae are roughed up and small strips of bone graft are placed over them. As this graft heals, the spine becomes solid and will not curve again.

A spinal fusion is typically performed in conjunction with insertion of a Harrington rod, a device that was developed by Paul Harrington, M.D., of Dallas, Texas. The Harrington rod has been used by surgeons for over 25 years in the correction of severe spinal deformities. During surgery, the surgeon places small hooks, which are attached to the rod, beneath the bones of the spine at the top and bottom of the curve along its inner (**concave**) side. The spine is straightened by jacking up the hooks on the rod, somewhat like lifting an automobile using a "bumper jack." The rod holds the spine as straight as possible while the spinal fusion heals.

The fusion is important because it makes the spine a solid continuous piece of bone. The rod is no longer essential once the spine completely heals, but usually is not removed unless problems occur. A cast or brace may be used to help hold the spinal correction and to protect the spine during healing. Wearing time for a cast or brace usually extends from 6 to 12 months following surgery.

If untreated, scoliosis may become more severe, causing permanent deformity of the spine and ribs. Ultimately, it may even interfere with breathing and heart functions.

Recommended Reading The Scoliosis Research Society has published a booklet, *Scoliosis: A Handbook for Patients,* to provide patients with a better understanding of the causes and treatment of scoliosis (Scoliosis Research Society, 1981). This most informative booklet focuses on idiopathic scoliosis and is recommended for all persons who are in contact with teenagers on an ongoing basis. It is available at nominal cost in quantities of 100 or more from the Scoliosis Research Society, 444 North Michigan Avenue, Chicago, Illinois 60611; phone: (312) 822-0970. Readers interested in a detailed description of scoliosis measurement, bracing, and surgical techniques should consider Dr. Rene Cailliet's book, *Scoliosis: Diagnosis and Management* (Cailliet, 1975). This reasonably priced book is an excellent introduction to the subject of scoliosis for both professionals and nonprofessionals.

When otherwise normal adolescents are treated for spinal curves, they are encouraged to participate actively in and cooperate with a treatment program. Young teenage girls with scoliosis might wish to place Judy Blume's book *Dennie* at the top of their reading list (Blume, 1973). The story, told from Dennie's viewpoint, expresses her worries about poor posture, doctor's examinations, the diagnosis of adolescent idiopathic scoliosis, and brace wearing. *Dennie* is also helpful for parents, teachers, therapists, doctors, and other adults who sometimes forget what it is like to be a teenager—especially a teenager dealing with a difficult problem.

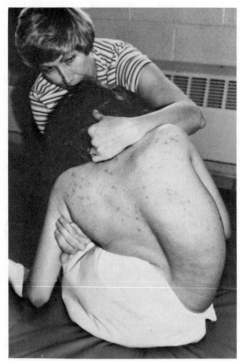

Figure 7.1. Severe scoliosis. Unfortunately, the patient in this photograph already had severe, untreated scoliosis when we first saw her 8 years ago. Note the rotation deformity of the spine in addition to the scoliosis (**rotoscoliosis**) that causes the rib cage to turn to the side. Her medical history indicates that she has been bedbound most of her life. She is unable to maintain a sitting position unassisted.

Scoliosis in Neuromuscularly and Severely Impaired Persons

The incidence of scoliosis among the neuromuscularly and severely involved population is much greater than among the general public. A 1973 study showed that 39% of severely involved institutionalized patients have scoliosis. Most of the worst curves are found in patients who have always been bedbound (Figure 7.1) (Samilson & Rechard, 1973). Furthermore, scoliosis found among those with neuromuscular involvement develops at a much earlier age than in the general population. This is due to the effects of brain damage upon the body, as discussed in Chapters 4 and 5. Therapists and doctors are alerted to the possible development of an abnormal spinal curve in brain damaged children by observing muscle tone and postural reflexes (see Chapter 10). Early detection and treatment of scoliosis is of utmost importance for all persons. However, prevention is a major goal of a physical management program for those with neuromuscular-related brain damage.

Scoliosis Development Scoliosis forms as an impaired child slumps more and more into a sideways leaning posture. At first, the curve can be straightened easily by holding the child in an upright position. If the problem goes untreated, however, the spinal curve increases and gradually becomes fixed and rigid as the child grows. As noted, idiopathic scoliosis in otherwise normal people takes place in the growth period of early teenage years. Brain damaged children also experience progression of the deformity during periods of rapid growth. However, because maturation is often delayed, growth spurts may continue into the late teen years or early twenties increasing the risk of severe curves (Fraser, Galka, & Hensinger, 1980). Parents and care providers will be the first to notice a child's growth spurts and should be particularly careful to maintain the child's torso in a straight position during these critical times.

Prevention and Treatment Scoliosis found in neuromuscularly and severely involved persons presents a more complicated problem for the patient, therapist, doctor, parents, and care providers than the idiopathic type of curve found in otherwise normal teenagers. Prevention becomes priority number one. Proper positioning is the cornerstone of a prevention program. At least in theory, it should be possible to prevent a severe deformity if enough attention can be paid to maintaining a sufficiently aligned posture to counteract the uneven pull of muscles caused by an individual's brain damage. Unfortunately, there has not been enough intensive work done with severely involved persons, nor enough research studies, to determine whether positioning theory carries over into achievable results for this population.

If scoliosis begins to develop despite the therapy received, emphasis shifts to aggressive treatment aimed at minimizing the deformity and, hopefully, keeping it from either interfering with daily activities or becoming life-threatening. Treatment may take a variety of forms depending upon the judgment of the attending physical therapist and orthopaedist. Treatment may include the use of

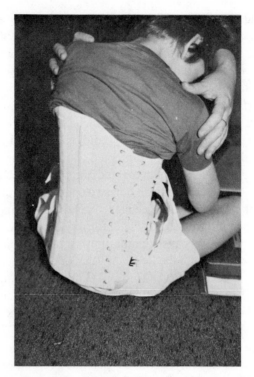

Figure 7.2. Canvas type corset. This 5-year-old boy has functional scoliosis. He wears the soft canvas corset to provide support for his spine when sitting and to prevent the functional scoliosis from becoming structural. Canvas type corsets are available from Freeman Manufacturing Co. and Medipedic Inc.

corsets, **orthoses,** wheelchair modifications, customized seating systems, wheelchair beds, therapeutic positioning, and surgery.

   Corsets   The authors suggest that a soft canvas-type corset may be used (Figure 7.2) for very young children, for persons with a mild deformity, and for those with severe deformities who cannot tolerate a more rigid type of support. The corset is worn all day over the person's undershirt. It is a prescriptive item and must be measured individually by a specialist for proper fitting (Figure 7.3). A larger one must be obtained to accommodate growth. The corset should be hand washed in lukewarm water with a mild soap and laid flat to dry. Drying time takes about two days. It is important that the corset be worn all day, every day. Therefore, two corsets should be ordered at a time so that one can be worn while the spare is washed. Since the

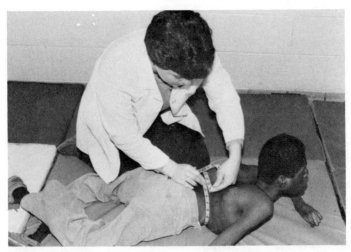

Figure 7.3. Measuring corset. An orthotist measures a student for a corset. The corset was prescribed at a school clinic. The orthotist comes to school to measure those who need corsets. She will also deliver the corset to school to show staff and parents exactly how to apply and remove it. This arrangement allows a student to attend school without interruption for visits to the hospital and orthotic store and provides opportunity to coordinate his equipment requirements with his family and teachers.

corset is worn outside an undershirt and is fairly soft, skin irritations are rare. However, it is important for care providers to remove the corset and check for skin redness at least twice a day.

A corset is easily applied and removed. In order to apply the corset, it is laid flat on a mat or bed with the inside facing upward. Next, the wearer is placed in a backlying (supine) position on top of the corset. Then, the front edges are brought around the wearer and fastened from bottom to top over the abdomen (Figure 7.4). This procedure helps to prevent the corset from riding upward. The corset should fit snug to the body, but not restrict breathing. It should be positioned so that there are two finger widths between the armpit and the top of the corset. In order to remove the corset, reverse the process described above.

A corset is designed to hold the handicapped person's torso in a straight position. While this may be somewhat restrictive to the person's active movement, it is a small price to pay for helping to minimize what could become a very serious deformity. Furthermore,

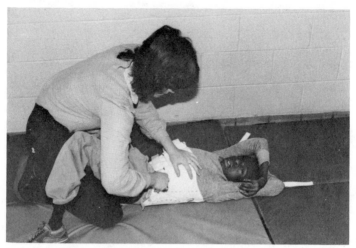

Figure 7.4. Fastening the corset. A teacher fastens the corset from bottom to top to prevent it from riding upward during the day's activities.

in most cases using a corset with severely impaired individuals actually improves gross motor ability because it holds the torso stabilized and permits more constructive use of arms and legs (Figure 7.5).

Orthoses Older children and patients with a moderate spinal deformity may require a support made from stronger material than canvas to hold their torsos in a straight position. Such a support is called an *orthosis*. Plastic (hard and soft) orthoses are used commonly for this purpose (Winter & Carlson, 1977). Hard plastic orthoses made in two pieces are called *clamshell* orthoses (Figure 7.6) because the pieces are made to fit together snugly much like a clam's shell when the two halves close. The clamshell design is inherently strong so it doesn't squeeze the chest or abdomen as much as the wrap-around jacket-type described later in this section. Therefore, it is preferable for persons with breathing problems and prominent breasts or abdomens.

Care providers often have problems when applying and handling this type of orthosis. Because the front and back pieces fit together so closely, it is easy to pinch a person's skin in the seams. Also, care must be taken to avoid placing the hard plastic orthosis

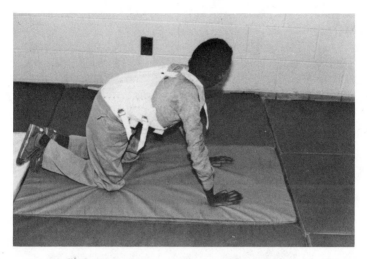

Figure 7.5. Corset enhances gross motor skill. After wearing his corset for a few days, this student learned to maintain this creeping position. The corset provided sufficient torso stability for him to forget about holding his torso steady and concentrate on constructive use of his arms and legs.

near a heat source such as a heat vent, stove, or direct sunlight. Excessive heat will cause the plastic to change shape.

Clamshell orthoses are made by a brace-maker (**orthotist**) who takes a plaster cast mold of the person's torso (referred to as a "negative" mold), much like the process used by doctors when setting a broken arm in a cast. The mold is cast in a position that at least partially corrects the person's spinal curve. Once the plaster hardens, it is removed from the patient and a plaster (positive) mold is made. The plastic is then molded over this positive plaster mold. Thus, the final hard plastic orthosis takes on every contour of the person's torso in the corrected position. Like the canvas corset, the clamshell orthosis is worn over the person's undershirt. Application is similar to that of the canvas corset. The back part of the clamshell is laid on the mat or bed. Then, the user, in a backlying position, is laid into the back piece. The front section is then placed carefully over the wearer's abdomen, and the two pieces are fastened into place. Unlike the corset, it is not necessary to begin fastening from the bottom up.

A one-piece soft plastic jacket orthosis (Figure 7.7) can be easier

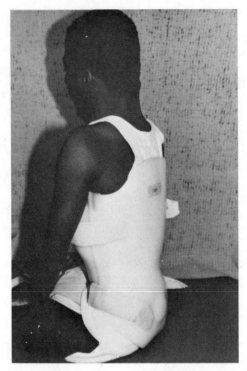

Figure 7.6. *Clamshell* orthosis. This two-piece orthosis is made of hard plastic. It is called a *clamshell* because the back and front fit together snugly much like a clam's shell when the two halves close.

for some attendants to apply and remove, causes less skin problems, and is more comfortable than the clamshell type. It, too, is constructed to fit the person by an orthotist. While a jacket type orthosis doesn't offer as much support as the hard plastic orthosis, it is considerably stronger than the canvas corset. Both the hard and soft plastic orthoses may cause skin irritations, and skin checks should be made at least twice a day. If redness is found, this should be reported to the supervising physical therapist who will coordinate any necessary modifications to the orthosis with the orthotist and orthopaedist.

Neuromuscularly and severely involved persons will need a build-up time when first wearing an orthosis. We recommend a skin check every hour for the first week and every 2 hours during the second week. Thereafter, a person may be able to tolerate the orthosis

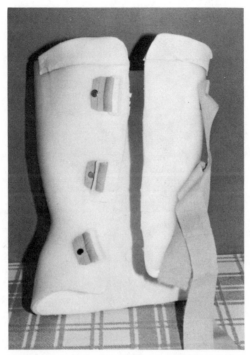

Figure 7.7. Jacket orthosis. This one-piece jacket-type orthosis is constructed of soft plastic. It is more comfortable for the patient and less troublesome to care providers than the clamshell type.

for several hours at a time. Skin checks should continue to be made twice a day after the break-in period. We do not encourage severely impaired patients to wear an orthosis during the night because staff are not available to monitor breathing. However, the attending therapist's and orthopaedist's instructions for a particular individual should be followed by care providers.

Wheelchair Modification　Another method of preventing and treating scoliosis in handicapped persons who lack sitting balance is to use a specially designed wheelchair that holds the person in a straight sitting position (Figure 7.8). The wheelchair must be carefully selected and fitted to the individual. Special attachments are added to position various parts of the person's body. Scoliosis pads are placed against the sides of the chest to prevent sideways leaning.

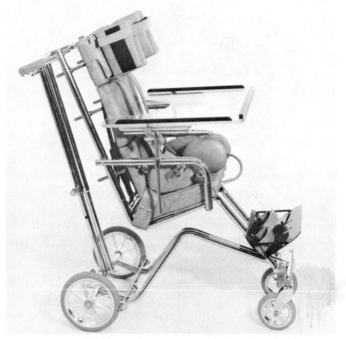

Figure 7.8.   Wheelchair modifications. This travel wheelchair is equipped with a head rest, harness, scoliosis pads, knee abductor, adjustable foot rest, and tray. It is available from Safety Travel Chairs, Inc. (Photograph courtesy of Safety Travel Chairs, Inc.)

An abductor pad may be placed between the knees to prevent crossing of the legs (**scissoring**) and to hold the person well back in the chair. Headrests are used to position the head so the person is looking straight ahead, and footrests are used to hold the feet at a right angle in a normal resting position. The handicapped person's position must be changed often. We recommend a 1-hour time limit between changes.

We prefer to keep nonwalking handicapped persons in commercially available wheelchairs as long as possible. These wheelchairs are less expensive than custom-made seating systems and most of them allow for adjustments to accommodate growth.

Customized Seating Systems   Teenage and adult neuromuscularly and severely involved persons often develop dislocations of the hip and contractures of pelvis muscles in addition to scoliosis (Rinsky & Kleinman, 1981). If the person becomes too deformed to use a commercially available wheelchair, customized seating systems can be employed. The systems are molded to the back and sides of the person's torso, hips, and thighs. The final mold is placed in a standard wheelchair frame. The purpose of such a seating system is to provide sitting comfort and to hold the person in a straighter body position than would be possible in other wheelchairs.

Customized seating systems are relatively new. Research on such seating systems is currently being conducted by various university rehabilitation engineering departments. A number of centers throughout the United States are involved in field testing and evaluation of these systems. It is likely that there will be a dramatic increase in the availability of customized seating systems in the next few years (Hobson, Driver, & Hanks, 1978).

Customized seating systems currently are of two types: seating orthoses and foam-in-place molds. Seating orthoses are constructed in the same way a clamshell or plastic jacket orthosis is made. An orthotist casts the person's back, buttocks, and thighs—usually with the patient lying over the edge of a table—to form a sitting mold

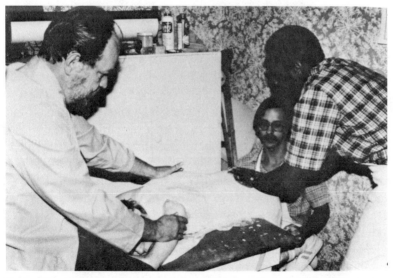

Figure 7.9. Construction of a seating orthosis. An orthotist and his assistants cast the back, buttocks, and thighs of the person lying over the edge of a table to form a sitting mold.

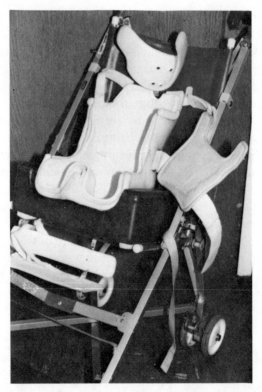

Figure 7.10. Seating orthosis. This orthosis was made by an orthotist to hold a particular student in a position that will partially correct a spinal curve.

(Figure 7.9). Partial correction of the spinal curve may be built into the mold by positioning the patient during the casting process. The hard plastic orthosis is inserted into a standard wheelchair frame to provide a firm support for the person's body (Figure 7.10).

The foam-in-place system consists of a soft foam which is molded to the person while in a sitting position (Figure 7.11). The foam, initially in a liquid form, expands to surround the back and sides of the person's head, torso, hips, and thighs. The soft foam mold is then covered with vinyl to protect the foam from urine and perspiration. The final product is attached to a wheelchair frame (Figure 7.12). Foam-in-place systems are used for persons with severe curves who cannot tolerate a rigid kind of correction. The

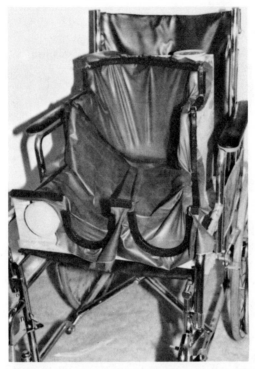

Figure 7.11. Foam-in-place frame. This wooden frame was made from measurements taken of a student's body. The liquid foam was poured into the capped areas at the bottom left and upper right of the frame while the person was sitting in the frame.

purpose of the foam-in-place, then, is to maintain the person in a comfortable sitting position and to prevent further deformity. Foam-in-place systems generally do not offer correction.

Care and maintenance of customized seats and management of the handicapped person are the same for both the orthosis and foam-in-place systems. The seat should be washed daily with a mild soap and water. Since both systems are closely molded to the body, the person should wear a light cotton shirt and trousers when using the seat. These systems are not designed to accommodate heavy or bulky clothes. In winter, a cape or blanket should be placed over the person and seat since coats and jackets cannot be worn while the person is in the seat.

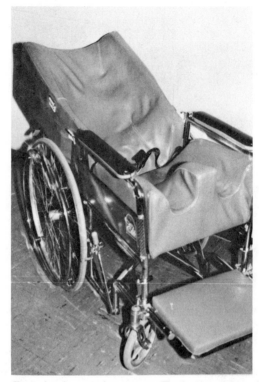

Figure 7.12. Foam-in-place seating system. The hardened foam is covered with vinyl and placed in a standard wheelchair frame. This foam-in-place seat was made for the person in Figure 7.1. This system holds her in a comfortable sitting position and allows her to be transported safely in a school bus. However, it offers little, if any, correction of her severe scoliosis.

Placing a severely deformed person in a customized seating system requires at least a two-person lift (see Chapter 12). The job will be easier if the chair (with the brakes locked) is tilted backward, resting against a table. This position allows gravity to help pull the person into the seat. Also, to ensure a proper seating position, the most deformed part of the person's body should be placed into the seat first.

Wheelchair Beds Persons with scoliosis who have lost the ability to sit, even in a totally supported position, may use a fully reclined wheelchair. In these cases of extreme deformity, bolsters are used in the chair to position the body in a comfortable position that

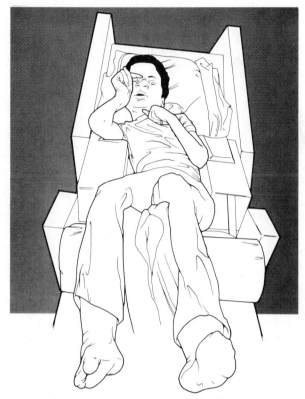

Figure 7.13. Positioning in a wheelchair bed. This illustration depicts a student with severe scoliosis. He is positioned with bolsters to assist his breathing.

allows for ease in breathing (Figure 7.13). Curves of the most severe nature compress vital organs within the chest and, thus, cause breathing and heart problems. At this point, correcting or limiting the progression of severe curves becomes secondary to the person's comfort. Attaching a photograph of the recommended position for a person on the back of his or her wheelchair can be very helpful. This approach is easier for others to understand than a set of involved written instructions.

Bed/mat Positioning　Since a handicapped person will not spend an entire day (hopefully) in a wheelchair, mat or bed positioning also is necessary. Three reclined positions may be used on a bed or mat: backlying (supine), facelying (prone), or sidelying. Since any movement of the head, arms, or legs may cause the torso of severely

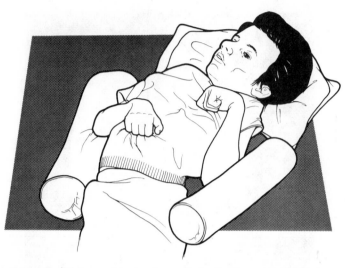

Figure 7.14. Backlying positioning for scoliosis. Sandbags are placed along both sides of this student's body to prevent his torso from curving to one side.

brain damaged persons to curve sideways, it often is necessary to use positioning aids such as bolsters, sandbags, and weights to keep the body straight (Galka, Fraser, & Hensinger, 1980).

In the backlying position, the person is placed on his or her back on a mat or bed, with a small pillow under the head and neck. Sandbags may be placed along both sides of the body to prevent the person's torso from curving to one side (Figure 7.14).

Obtaining a straight facelying position is a bit more complicated. Placing a severely impaired person flat on a bed or mat requires that the face be turned to one side. This may make it difficult to keep the torso from curving. We suggest placing the person's chest over a bolster or small wedge with the forehead resting upon another bolster or towel (see Figure 10.15). This will keep the head from turning and allow for easy breathing. Another small towel roll may be placed under the ankles to prevent the legs from turning and to keep pressure off the toes. Again, sandbags may be placed against each side of the body to keep the torso from curving.

Commercially made sidelying boxes are available to support a handicapped person in a straight sidelying position (see Figure 10.16). If such a box is not available, the person may be held in a sidelying position by using pillows or bolsters placed against the front and back of the torso. The pillows or bolsters may be anchored using sandbags if necessary.

It is important that care providers watch a handicapped person closely during positioning. Remove the person from the position at once if he or she shows signs of distress.

Surgical Treatment   With present spinal instrumentation (such as the Harrington rod), it is possible to correct, or at least stabilize, most spinal deformities that occur in neuromuscularly and severely impaired persons. However, such surgery involves many risks and complications and requires prolonged periods of hospitalization and time in body casts. Such experiences are physically demanding on a handicapped person. Problems with drooling and lack of bowel and bladder control make it particularly difficult for a severely impaired person's skin to tolerate postoperative casting (Rinsky & Kleinman, 1981). Whenever possible, we prefer to modify standard procedures so that the individual has the shortest possible period of immobilization, spends less time in casts, and has the shortest practicable cast to reduce the chance of pressure sores (**decubitus ulcers**) (Fraser et al., 1980).

An interesting new development for neuromuscularly and severely impaired persons is the Luque instrumentation devised by Eduardo Luque, M.D., of Mexico City. This system, which was used initially in patients with polio, features one or two rods wired directly to the spine. (Sometimes, it is referred to as an intersegmental instrumentation since each vertebra is fixed to the rod.) The system provides much firmer fixation to the spine than surgeons are able to obtain with the two-hook method of the Harrington rod.

The Luque instrumentation is particularly appropriate for neuromuscularly and severely impaired persons since a firm external control, such as a cast, is not required following the procedure. Some patients may need only a brace after such surgery; others will require no external support whatsoever. The absence of casting is of great benefit to neuromuscularly and severely impaired persons, most of whom have difficulty tolerating casts, and to their care providers in attending to postoperative hygiene needs.

A drawback of the Luque procedure is that the attaching wires have to pass under the thin, flat plate (**laminae**) of the vertebrae into

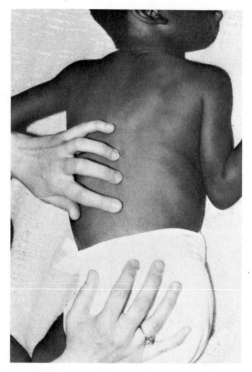

Figure 7.15. Mild scoliosis. The child in this photograph has a slight C-shaped sideways curvature of the spine. This curve is illustrated by the fingers touching over the spinous processes.

the spinal canal and back out again. Thus, there is potential risk of neurological injury. The surgeon, patient, and family should discuss the risks in detail and weigh those versus the benefits of the procedure.

With handicapped persons, a decision for surgery is based mainly on anticipated functional gain (Rinsky & Kleinman, 1981). By this we mean the extent to which the person may be expected to exhibit improved gross motor ability as a result of the surgery. The surgeon must balance the relative risk of surgery versus the gain in function or in prevention of a progressively more severe deformity. Since parents and care providers know the handicapped person best, they can provide information that will help the surgeon weigh the pros (gains) and cons (risks) of operating. For example, the surgeon may want to know if the person is experiencing pain. If so, is the pain severe enough to warrant surgical correction? Is the procedure being considered reliable for pain relief? Would an individual use his or her hands purposefully if they weren't needed for support when sitting? Is it becoming more difficult to lift or dress the person? Will he or she be able to cooperate with postoperative care? Will he or she be motivated to improve in function following a surgical correction? Will further progression of the deformity limit cardiopulmonary function, ability to sit, stand, and so on? All of these questions can be answered best by those who are around the impaired person every day.

Surgery is usually not considered when the curve is mild, that is, when it is between 20 and 40 degrees (Figure 7.15). However, it is important for parents to realize that the best surgical results are obtained while the scoliosis is still moderate (40–60 degrees) (Figure 7.16). Parents are often apprehensive about putting a child through

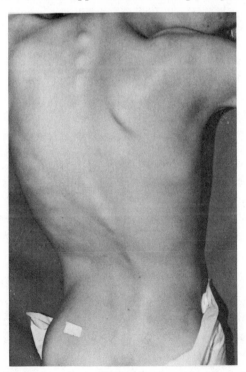

Figure 7.16. Moderate scoliosis. This student has a double, or S-shaped curve.

surgery when the spinal curve is moderate and not obviously deforming in appearance. However, the surgeon can obtain a much better
correction at less risk to the patient if surgery is performed before the
curve develops into a severe and rigid state (see Figure 7.1). Therefore, if surgery is inevitable (the curve is documented by X ray as
being progressive and cannot be controlled by conservative techniques such as braces and positioning), the decision should be made
at a time when the curve is moderate, and not postponed until later
when the risks increase and the results are likely to be poorer.

If surgery is decided upon, close cooperation between the
hospital staff and those familiar with an impaired individual's routine
is essential. A severely impaired patient, in particular, can pose
unique problems for the hospital staff in communication, feeding,
and personal care. We recommend that a comprehensive report about
the student from the school staff or parents be sent to the surgeon
when the person enters the hospital. This information is shared with
the nursing staff, who can plan accordingly.

It is important that the patient remain as functional as possible
following surgery and return as quickly as possible to a normal
routine. Follow-up care after discharge should be discussed before
admission to the hospital so that all concerned can be aware of care
requirements during the recovery and rehabilitation period. Those
caring for the patient should watch postsurgical progress closely, and
any problems should be reported to the surgeon. If potential problems
are left unchecked, surgical benefits may be lost, and the person's
condition might even regress. The parents' understanding and cooperation, along with that of care providers, is vital to successful
surgical treatment of scoliosis. It is equally true for other types of
surgery (as described in Chapters 8 and 9) that the handicapped
person may encounter.

ABNORMAL LORDOSIS AND KYPHOSIS

Abnormal forward and backward curvatures of the spine often are
found in neuromuscularly and severely involved persons, as well as
among the normal population. These curves are less of a problem to
the handicapped person and to care providers than scoliosis, and

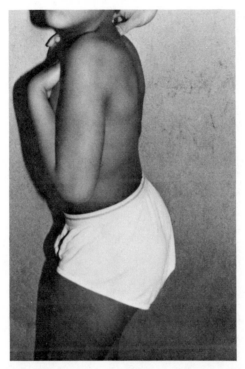

Figure 7.17. Lordosis. This person has a slight forward curve of his lower spine. A lordosis is sometimes referred to as a "hollow back" or "sway back."

usually are not life-threatening. Lordosis and kyphosis, however, may be found commonly in combination with scoliosis.

Normal people who have a pathological lordosis (Figure 7.17) and/or kyphosis (Figure 7.18) are considered to have poor posture. Physical therapists prescribe exercises to improve this type of back problem. In many cases, neuromuscularly involved persons also can benefit from such an exercise program, but most severely impaired persons cannot exercise. Therefore, positioning and supports are used to control the problem and make such persons comfortable (Galka, Fraser, & Hensinger, 1980). For wheelchair-bound persons with lordosis, a small pillow or foam can be placed behind the low back for support and for prevention of discomfort from back strain. For persons with severe kyphosis (Figure 7.19), a soft plastic orthosis

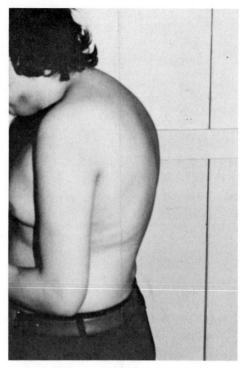

Figure 7.18. Kyphosis. The person pictured has a backward curve of the upper spine. The kyphosis causes a hump-like appearance of the back.

jacket may be prescribed to support the back and help the person to maintain an upright sitting posture (Figure 7.20). Surgical correction is seldom necessary for lordosis and kyphosis when found in neuro-muscularly and severely involved persons.

OPISTHOTONOS

In rare instances involving severely impaired persons, severe muscle spasms cause the spine to extend completely so that a person is bent backward like a bow (Figure 7.21). Such extreme cases defy attempts to position the body. Therefore, medication is used as the first level of treatment to reduce the spasms. Once the spasms are under control, therapeutic positioning is resumed. Opisthotonos is a life-threatening

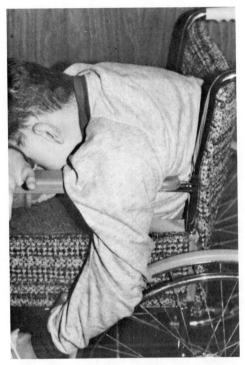

Figure 7.19. Severe kyphosis. This student has a severe backward curve of the upper spine that causes him to fall forward in his wheelchair.

condition because extreme hyperextension of the head makes it difficult for an affected person to swallow.

CONCLUSION

Doctors and therapists only direct the team effort aimed at preventing and treating spinal deformities in neuromuscularly and severely involved persons. It is the day-to-day handling of these individuals by parents and care providers that may make the difference between a person's maintaining a relatively normal looking body or developing a serious deformity.

However, it is important that both parents and care providers realize that spinal deformities may develop despite the best efforts of

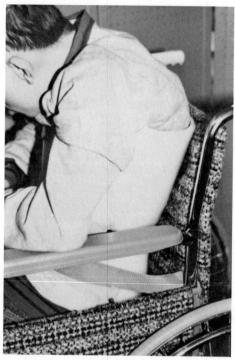

Figure 7.20. Jacket orthosis for kyphosis. The student shown in Figure 7.19 uses a soft plastic orthosis (see Figure 7.7) when he sits in his wheelchair. It is comfortable for him and is easily removed by care providers when he is on the floor mat.

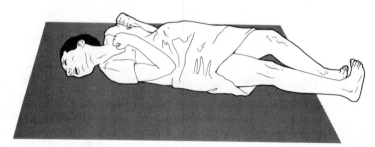

Figure 7.21. Opisthotonos. The severely impaired person in this illustration is bent backward like a bow due to severe muscle spasms. Opisthotonos is life-threatening because extreme hyperextension of the head makes it difficult to swallow food.

all concerned to prevent them. If this occurs, it should be accepted as a result of the handicapped person's brain damage and not blamed on failure to provide proper care. Continued efforts should always be made to arrest progression of the deformity.

REFERENCES

Blume, J. *Dennie* New York: Dell Publishing Company, 1973.

Cailliet, R. *Scoliosis: Diagnosis and management.* Philadelphia: F.A. Davis Co., 1975.

Fraser, B.A., Galka, G., & Hensinger, R.N. *Gross motor management of severely multiply impaired students, Vol. I: Evaluation guide.* Baltimore: University Park Press, 1980.

Galka, G., Fraser, B.A., & Hensinger, R.N. *Gross motor management of severely impaired students, Vol. II: Curriculum model.* Baltimore: University Park Press, 1980.

Hobson, D., Driver, K.D., & Hanks, S. *Foam-in-place seating for the severely disabled: Preliminary results.* Paper presented at the Interagency Conference on Rehabilitation Engineering, Washington, DC, September, 1978.

Rinsky, L.A., & Kleinman, R.G. Surgical treatment of scoliosis in cerebral palsy. *American Academy of Cerebral Palsy and Developmental Medicine News,* 1981, *101*(32), 1–3.

Samilson, R.L., & Rechard, R. Scoliosis in cerebral palsy. Incidence, distribution of curve patterns, natural history and thoughts on etiology. *Current Practices in Orthopaedic Surgery,* 1973, *5*, 183–205.

Scoliosis Research Society. *Scoliosis: A handbook for patients.* Chicago: Scoliosis Research Society, 1981.

Winter, R.B., & Carlson, J.M. Modern orthotics for spinal deformities. *Clinical Orthopaedics and Related Research,* 1977, *126*, 74–86.

Deformities of the Arms and Hands

8

Deformities of the arms and hands (upper extremities) are quite common among persons with neuromuscular involvement, and particularly among severely impaired individuals. Their occurrence in the arms and hands differs from lower extremity involvement (see Chapter 9) in that deformities tend to be more severe when located further away from the trunk. Thus, such deformities occur least commonly in the shoulder, somewhat more frequently in the elbow, and most often in the wrist and hand. Typically, upper extremity deformities occur in combination.

For the normal person, the hands may be viewed as an extension of the mind, allowing performance of self-care, feeding, work, and recreational activities. At least minimal use of the arms and hands is of great benefit to severely impaired persons. For example, nonverbal persons often use their hands as a way of communicating (see Chapter 11). Being able to hold a toy is a source of interest and comfort to many severely mentally and physically impaired individuals. Thus, it is important that hand function in physically impaired persons be maintained and, when possible, improved.

Arm and hand deformities usually do not contribute to postural deformities of the spine as is true of many deformities of the lower extremities. As such, arm and hand deformities generally do not produce serious, sometimes life-threatening complications.

SHOULDER DEFORMITIES

In most neuromuscularly and severely involved persons, shoulders usually do not show obvious deformities (Keats, 1970). Looks may be deceiving, however, and often the shoulder may be stiff and joint mobility (range of motion) may be restricted. Less commonly, the shoulder joints of some neuromuscularly and severely involved persons may be abnormally loose and, in rare cases, may dislocate. To reduce the possibility of further damage to shoulder joints, care providers should be cautious about pulling physically impaired persons by the arms. It is safer to shift his or her position by reaching behind the back and pulling the upper torso forward.

Care providers also should be aware that it is easy to fracture the upper arm bone **(humerus)** of an impaired person by squeezing or pulling. It is wise to avoid restraining an impaired person by the arms.

ELBOW AND FOREARM DEFORMITIES

Abnormal joint flexion is the most common elbow and forearm deformity found among neuromuscularly and severely involved persons. It is produced by contractures of the muscles that bend the elbow and turn the forearm in a palm down position (pronation) (see Figure 8.1). This type of deformity is experienced in the involved arm by many cerebral palsied patients, particularly those with spastic hemiplegia, and in both arms by most severely impaired persons (Keats, 1970).

Persons with only a slight flexion contracture of the elbow experience little inconvenience. However, much like spinal deformities such as scoliosis, elbow flexion deformity is progressive and tends to worsen during periods of growth (Bleck, 1979). Care providers should be certain that the attending therapist is aware of an increasing contracture so that preventive measures such as splints and positioning may be prescribed. Without preventive measures, some

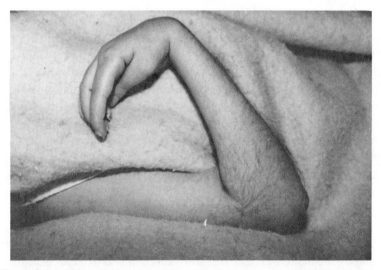

Figure 8.1. Elbow flexion deformity. This photo shows the maximum extent to which this elbow joint can be straightened. For the first several years of life, this individual had normal range of motion in the elbow joint. As time passed, brain damage caused a muscle imbalance to develop in the muscles controlling elbow movement. The eventual result was this elbow deformity.

individuals eventually may develop such a severe contracture that they lose all ability to extend the elbow.

In the case of individuals who already have a badly contracted elbow, there is danger of skin breakdown in the elbow crease. Elbow protectors for persons with severe elbow flexion contractures may help to prevent breakdown of the skin around the elbow.

Care providers are likely to experience difficulty dressing individuals who have a moderate to severe degree of elbow contracture. To minimize the problem of putting on a coat or shirt, place the most deformed arm in a sleeve first. When removing the garment, take the most deformed arm out last (Finnie, 1975). By following this pattern, less strain will be placed on the deformed arm, the job will be easier, and the process will be more comfortable for the physically impaired person.

Surgical Treatment

Surgery usually is not considered in cases of elbow flexion contracture where there are only slight restrictions in motion and function. Instead, continuing therapy is employed to maintain the existing range of motion. However, if the deformity causes problems for the individual and for care providers, surgical release of the tight muscles at the elbow may be helpful to improve extension and, in some instances, improve hand function (Bleck, 1979). Presently, surgery for the elbow is limited to simple soft tissue procedures designed to lengthen the muscles that bend the elbow. These surgical procedures place the elbow in a more extended position. Unfortunately, they may not result in improved elbow function. Even so, the placement of the elbow in extension may let the person perform hand activities away from the body such as reaching for a toy or cup placed on a tray or table.

If surgery is performed, a postoperative exercise program is essential to maintaining the flexibility and extension that has been gained. In such cases, the attending surgeon and occupational therapist will prescribe an appropriate program that may involve exercise activities and splinting.

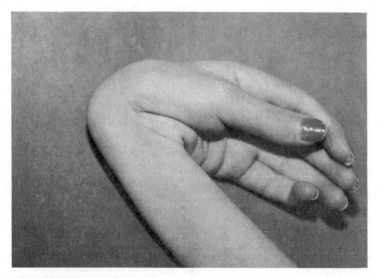

Figure 8.2. Wrist flexion—ulnar deviation deformity. This is a common type of wrist deformity in which the wrist assumes a flexed position and the hand turns sideways.

WRIST DEFORMITIES

In the most common type of wrist deformity, the wrist assumes a flexed position and the hand deviates to one side (ulnar deviation) (Figure 8.2). Splints may be used to hold the wrist and hand in a more functional position (Figure 8.3) (Malick, 1972). This deformity presents few problems to care providers in terms of cleansing and dressing the person. However, if the deformity becomes severe, it may limit hand function and make dressing difficult. A wrist deformity usually is not painful to a neuromuscularly or severely involved person, although occasionally such persons may complain of pain in the wrist. While surgery usually isn't necessary to relieve pain, it may be considered for cosmetic and convenience reasons.

Surgical Treatment

A wrist fusion (**arthrodesis)** is an operation that makes the wrist permanently stiff. Wrist fusions have become increasing popular for handicapped teenagers who are concerned about appearance. The

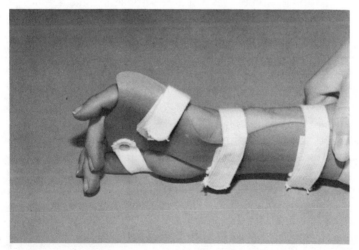

Figure 8.3. Splint for wrist flexion—ulnar deviation wrist deformity. An occupational therapist designed and fabricated this splint for a student who showed signs of developing a wrist deformity such as the one pictured in Figure 8.2. Notice that the splint is designed to hold the wrist in extension and prevent the hand from drifting sideways.

wrist fusion makes the wrist and hand appear more normal. This operation is particularly effective for a hemiplegic person who has a deformed wrist and hand that are not very functional. Many hemiplegic persons use the nonfunctional hand to stabilize a book, paper, plate, or object upon which they are working. The fused wrist works as a more efficient stabilizer than a badly deformed wrist and makes the handicap less noticeable as well. It also allows a shirt or coat to be put on more quickly.

For carefully selected persons, tendon transfers (a soft tissue procedure) may help to position the wrist in a neutral or more functional position. However, tendon transfers about the wrist have met with limited success in neuromuscularly and severely impaired persons due to the lack of voluntary control over the muscles that move the wrist.

HAND DEFORMITIES

Hand deformities, as they progress, may reach a point where they interfere with and sometimes prohibit purposeful hand activity. This is true even for severely impaired persons who have lost their muscle coordination through brain damage. Hand deformities are conspicuous and can be a source of embarassment for an impaired person. Occupational therapists place special emphasis on treating these deformities. For example, they may design special hand grips to help impaired persons grasp objects. Handgrips may be added to a bike to allow a hemiplegic person to keep both hands on the bike's handlebars and thus improve weight distribution and riding balance. It should be noted that special wheelchair adaptations, such as a one-arm drive on a standard wheelchair and controls for either a right or left hand on a power chair, are available for persons with only one functional hand (see Chapter 13).

Thumb-in-Hand Deformity

This deformity's name describes the position assumed by the thumb, which becomes tightly bent into the palm of the hand in a flexed position. Such a deformity limits grasp and pinch movements needed to hold objects. In severely impaired persons, care providers may find that the position of the thumb makes it difficult to clean an affected person's hand completely. It is better to soak the hand in

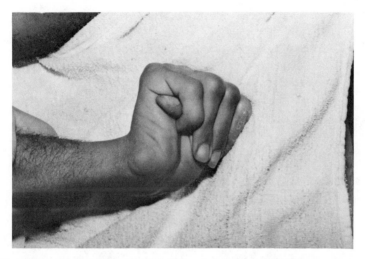

Figure 8.4.   Severe thumb-in-palm deformity. The deformity's name describes the position assumed by the thumb. In this case, the fingers have flexed over the thumb compounding the problem. Care providers find it very difficult to clean a hand like this completely.

soapy water than to forcibly pry the thumb away from the palm in order to clean under it with a washcloth.

Often, the fingers flex over the thumb, compounding the problem (Figure 8.4). Where this condition is present, gently bending the wrist by pushing on the back of the hand will extend the fingers. They will open naturally (Figure 8.5). Do not pry the fingers open to wash the hand and fingers (Figure 8.6). This will only cause them to tighten even more around the thumb. If the thumb is flexible, splints may be used to hold the thumb away from the palm to prevent further deformity (Figure 8.7) (Cailliet, 1975). Splints are custom-made by an occupational therapist, who also assigns wearing schedules. In cold climates, mittens may be placed over a person's hand while a splint is being used. Mittens should be worn by impaired individuals, particularly those who suck their fingers or thumbs, when outside in cold weather to avoid frostbite. Gloves, of course, cannot be worn.

Finger Flexion Deformity

When this deformity is present, the fingers flex into the palm of the hand. The thumb, however, remains outside the palm in a relatively normal resting position. Again, the major problem for care providers

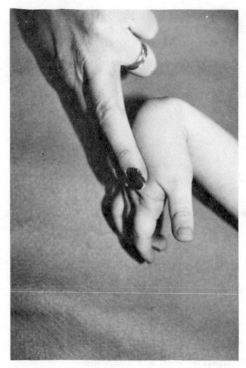

Figure 8.5. Correct way to extend fingers in a severe thumb-in-palm deformity. Gently push on the back of the hand, bending the wrist, in order to extend the fingers and bring the thumb away from the hand.

is cleansing the hand. The same procedure should be used as was discussed in connection with the palm-in-hand deformity—gentle pressure on the back of the hand—to open the fingers. An affected person's fingernails should be clipped very short and cut regularly to prevent injury to the skin from sharp nails. The attending occupational therapist may design a splint to hold the fingers in a more extended position (Figure 8.8) or use a cone (Figure 8.9) for the same purpose (Malick, 1972).

Surgical Treatment of the Thumb and Fingers

With hand deformities, the most common reasons for surgery are to improve hand function, appearance, and hygiene (Bleck, 1979). Surgical procedures for neuromuscularly and severely involved per-

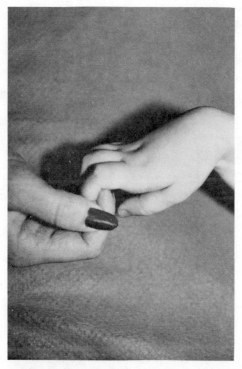

Figure 8.6. Incorrect way to extend fingers in a severe thumb-in-palm deformity. Do not pry the fingers open. This will cause them to flex tighter. Compare the position of the thumb with the photo of the same hand in Figure 8.5. Bending the wrist by pushing on the back of the hand causes the thumb to naturally spread away from the hand.

sons include release, transfer, and lengthening of involved tendons, as well as joint fusions. Simple surgical procedures, such as tendon lengthenings, are usually able to relax muscle pull and release the fingers and thumb from the palm. Stabilization procedures (bony surgery) that fix the thumb in a better position can be helpful with carefully selected patients.

For the mildly involved person, additional procedures may be considered to permit finer movement and to improve function. For example, a procedure that widens the web space between the index finger and the thumb is effective in permitting a larger grasp and allowing the thumb to be brought out of the palm for pinch and grasp.

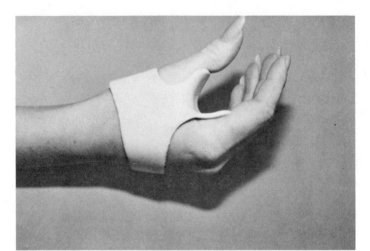

Figure 8.7. Thumb abduction splint. This splint is designed to hold the thumb away from the palm of the hand.

A postoperative program, planned jointly by the surgeon and occupational therapist, is important to maintaining the flexibility that has been gained and assisting the person to develop additional function. Parents and care providers can be of great assistance to the

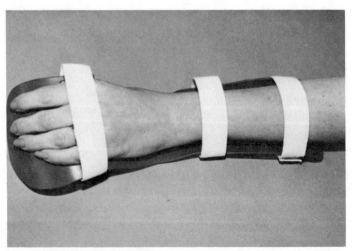

Figure 8.8. Resting pan splint. This type of splint is molded to the individual's hand to hold the fingers in a more extended and functional position.

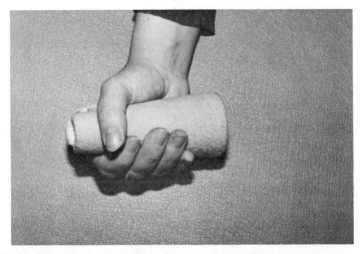

Figure 8.9. Hand cone. Like the finger extension splint, the hand cone is used to hold the fingers in a more extended position and prevent finger flexion deformities. However, the hand cone usually is not a custom-made splint. One size fits all hands. Note that the small end of the cone is placed between the thumb and index finger with the large end of the cone resting in the palm at the little finger side of the hand. Hand cones may be purchased from T.J. Posy Company and Fred Sammons, Inc.

surgeon and occupational therapist in evaluating a physically impaired person's needs and in planning pre- and postoperative care.

Recommended Reading If hand surgery is contemplated, we suggest that the reader refer to Dr. Eugene Bleck's book *Orthopaedic Management of Cerebral Palsy* (Bleck, 1979). The chapter on spastic hemiplegia contains excellent illustrations of various hand surgical procedures. Although this book is geared toward the health professional, lay readers interested in hand surgical techniques will find it helpful. Some might wish to use it in discussions with the attending orthopaedist or occupational therapist.

REFERENCES

Bleck, E.E. *Orthopaedic management of cerebral palsy. Saunders Monographs in Clinical Orthopaedics*, Vol. 2. Philadelphia: W.B. Saunders Co. 1979.

Cailliet, R. *Hand pain and impairment*. Philadelphia: F.A. Davis Company, 1975.

Finnie, N.R. *Handling the young cerebral palsied child at home*. New York: E.F. Dutton & Co., 1975.

Keats, S. *Operative orthopedics in cerebral palsy.* Springfield, IL: Charles C Thomas, 1970.

Malick, M.H. *Manual on static hand splinting: New materials and techniques.* Pittsburgh: Harmarville Rehabilitation Center, 1972.

Deformities of the Legs and Feet

9

Deformities of the hips, legs, and feet (lower extremities) present more problems to both neuromuscularly and severely involved persons and care providers than deformities of the upper extremities. Hip deformities are particularly serious because they may cause pain, disturb the balance of the pelvis, and contribute to the development of scoliosis. Knee and foot deformities may interfere with standing balance. This chapter examines deformities of the leg separately, starting with the hip and working down to the feet. However, it is important to note that deformities of the hips, legs, and feet almost always coexist (Bleck, 1979a).

HIP DEFORMITIES

Hip deformities are a common cause of serious posture problems in neuromuscularly and severely involved persons. The pelvis and hips are the base upon which the spine is built. If the base is not straight and symmetrical, the spinal column will become unbalanced, which in turn may lead to spinal deformities (see Chapter 7). This discussion of hip deformities focuses on hip dislocations, **subluxations,** extension deformities, and abduction-flexion deformities, inasmuch as these are the principal conditions likely to be encountered with neuromuscularly and severely involved persons.

Hip Dislocations and Subluxations

Parents and care providers often express dismay upon learning that a neuromuscularly or severely involved child or adolescent has a dislocated hip. Such a reaction is understandable, but it results in part from confusion between a *dislocation* and a **fracture.** A dislocation of the hip joint occurs when the top (head) of the thigh bone (femur) separates from the hip socket (acetabulum). The dislocations that occur in neuromuscularly and severely impaired persons are not the kind of acute, sudden, violent phenomena that can happen to otherwise normal people in motorcycle or automobile accidents. Hip dislocations in neuromuscularly and severely impaired persons typically involve a slow, progressive deformation of the joint. The joint deforms over a long period of time, usually years, with the femoral head gradually working its way out of the socket. While a hip dislocation can be serious, it does not require emergency medical treatment as would a fracture.

Breaking of bones (fracture) is not a common problem for neuromuscularly and severely involved persons because muscle spasticity puts extra stress on bones, tending to strengthen them and make them more resistant to fracture. Conversely, persons who are paralyzed or who have extremities with little or no muscle power have very thin bones that fracture easily. There are also certain congenital conditions, such as osteogenesis imperfecta, that prevent the body from making firm or thick bones. As mentioned in Chapter 4, care providers must be especially careful when handling persons who have thin bones. Special caution must be used in positioning their legs, particularly if contractures or tightness about the hips and knees are present that prevent the legs from moving freely. When placing such a person in a chair or in bed it is comparatively easy to cause a fracture.

Most persons with neuromuscular involvement, including those who are severely impaired, are born with normal hip joints. Deformity, however, occurs during the growth process (Bleck, 1979b). In the case of cerebral palsied and severely impaired persons, spastic unbalanced muscle forces gradually deform bones and joints that were normal at birth. As mentioned previously, a hip dislocation does not happen suddenly because the head of the femur "jumps" out of its socket. Instead, the femoral head slowly "grows" out of the socket because of abnormal muscle forces across the joint. This process starts with normal hip joints (Figure 9.1a); then, over time, a small separation (subluxation) of the bones occurs (Figure 9.1b) and eventually develops into a dislocation (Figure 9.1c).

Dislocations of the hip occur frequently in neuromuscularly and severely impaired persons. In fact, they are so common among the severely impaired population that *all* such persons should be considered at risk (Fraser, Galka, & Hensinger, 1980). It is important that those involved in caring for severely impaired young children be alert to early symptoms of dislocation.

A child beginning to pull or scissor his or her legs tightly together (see Figure 10.10) is often the first sign of impending dislocation. This is caused by spasticity of the thigh muscles (**hip adductors**). At this stage, X rays may show a hip subluxation. (Methods of handling this type of problem are discussed in Chapter 10). As a hip dislocation develops—usually by age 7—one leg will appear shorter than the other (Figure 9.2) (Samilson, Tsov, Aamoth, & Green, 1972). If an affected individual lies on his or her back with knees bent, a dislocated hip will cause one knee to be at a different level than the other one.

A dislocated hip can disturb the balance of the pelvis (pelvic obliquity), leading to unequal pressure over the buttocks when sitting. This increases the potential for formation of bed sores (decubiti) and scoliosis (Fraser et al., 1980).

Dislocated hips are usually not painful at first, but they may become so. In a study of institutionalized cerebral palsy patients with hip dislocation, pain was found to be present in about half. In most cases, the pain was mild. However, just under 10% experienced severe pain (Moreau, Drummond, Rogala, Asworth, & Porter, 1978). Pain tends to occur in more neurologically aware or higher functioning individuals, especially in the person with the athotoid type of cerebral palsy.

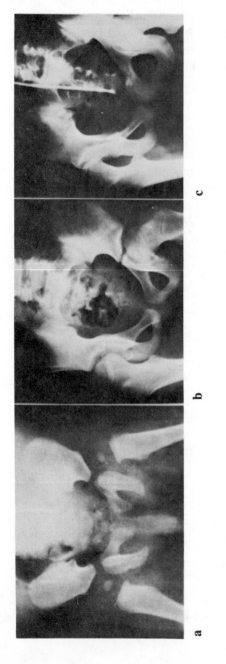

a

b

c

Figure 9.1. Process of hip dislocation. **a)** Normal X-ray (roentgenographic) appearance of the hips. This X ray is of an 8-month-old cerebral palsied girl with spastic muscle involvement on the right side of her body. The X-ray appearance of the hips is normal at this early age. Note that both hips appear symmetrical, and the pelvis is level. **b)** Subluxation of right hip. An X ray of the same child at age 5 shows evidence of a right hip subluxation. Note that the head of the femur (thigh bone) has risen upward in the hip socket (acetabulum), caused by the unbalanced pull of the spastic hip adductor muscles on the right leg. The acetabulum has developed abnormally (acetabular **dysplasia**) in response to the position of the femoral head. **c)** Dislocated right hip. By age 13 the girl's right hip has become dislocated. Note that the head of the right femur is now almost completely out of the acetabulum, which is misshapen. The pelvis is tilted (pelvic obliquity). The progression shown in these X rays is typical of hip deformities in brain damaged children. Bones and joints are normal at birth. With growth, the influence of the abnormal spastic muscles, *if untreated*, may lead to subluxation and subsequent dislocation of the hip.

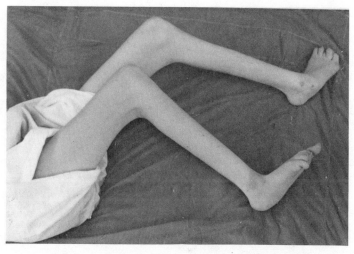

Figure 9.2.   Dislocated hip causes leg to appear shorter. The teenager in this photo has a dislocated right hip. Because the femur rides up and out of the acetabulum, her right leg appears shorter than the left and her right knee is at a lower level than the left knee.

Management of Hip Dislocations   A question often asked by both parents and care providers is whether a person with a dislocated hip should be placed in a standing position. We would discourage this activity *only* if the person shows signs of pain while standing or walking. Normally, a standing position will not aggravate a dislocated hip.

The continuous tension of scissoring legs is far more harmful to the hip joint than standing or walking (Fraser et al., 1980). Therefore, it is important to separate the legs while an individual is resting in bed or in a chair. When the person is in a backlying, facelying, or sidelying position, a hard bolster (do not use a spongy material) or towel roll should be placed between the thighs to hold the legs apart (Figure 9.3). Most wheelchairs and infant seats (see Chapter 13) made for handicapped children have an abductor pad to keep the legs separated.

Surgical Treatment   Surgical release of thigh adductor muscles or tendon transfer are often considered when the hip is in the early stages of deforming and only subluxed (Fraser et al., 1980). This is a soft tissue surgical procedure that involves cutting muscles,

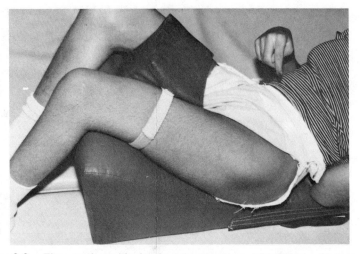

Figure 9.3. Therapeutic positioning for scissoring legs. A hard bolster (abductor wedge) is placed between this student's thighs to hold her legs apart, and an inclined wedge is placed under her thighs to hold her hips in a flexed position. Both the abductor wedge and inclined wedge are available from J. A. Preston Corp.

not bone. The surgery is referred to as "adductor release" because the surgeon cuts or sections the tendon or tendons of the hip adductor muscles. (The hip adductor muscle group consists of long and short muscles.) In performing the surgery, the surgeon usually cuts the long adductor muscle, which in most people can be felt under the skin in the groin area, and reattaches the tendon to lessen its pull. If the adductor muscle group is particularly spastic, one of the branches of the **obturator nerve** that goes into the muscle mass may be cut. Cutting this nerve decreases the force of the adductor muscle contraction. In cases where the adductor muscles are extremely tight, some of the short adductor muscles also may be lengthened. Depending upon the individual case, the surgeon may lengthen or transfer other tendons about the hip. It is important that the surgeon not over-release the adductor muscles. If this should occur, the person may develop an abduction deformity that may be more troublesome than the subluxed hip.

The surgical scar for an adductor release is located in the groin area (Figure 9.4). Following surgery, the patient usually is placed in a simple abduction cast or brace to hold the legs apart for the first few

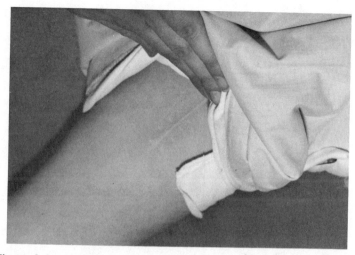

Figure 9.4. Surgical scar from adductor release. The surgical scar from an adductor release is only a few inches long and occurs high on the inside of the leg near the groin. The photograph shows a recent scar that will fade with time. An adductor release scar may become hidden in the fold of groin skin and often will be noticed only upon close inspection.

weeks of healing, and then is started on a vigorous exercise program to maintain the surgical correction.

The goal of such surgery is to prevent dislocations and, in the case of severely impaired individuals, to make it easier for care providers to change diapers and keep the diaper area clean. Soft tissue procedures, such as the hip adductor release, are not complex, require a fairly short operating time, and are much less demanding on the patient than more complicated bony surgery.

Once the hip becomes dislocated, surgery involving the hip bones is needed to correct the dislocation (Fraser et al., 1980). These procedures are technically difficult and more prone to problems such as stiffness of the joint than soft tissue surgery. Also, the recovery period for bony surgery is considerably longer than for soft tissue surgery.

Unfortunately, for many neuromuscularly and severely impaired persons, the dislocation has developed over a long time period, and thus many adaptive changes have taken place in the joint. An extensive surgical procedure is required to place the head of the

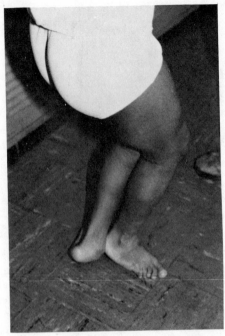

Figure 9.5. Tight hip adductor muscles cause loss of walking balance. The student in this photograph experienced a significant tightening of both hip adductor muscles at age 12. The muscle tightness became so severe that she lost the ability to walk and to separate her legs.

femur into the socket (reduce the hip). Often, the socket needs to be reconstructed to permit the femoral head to be replaced in the joint. This entails a complex procedure involving both the proximal femur and the acetabulum. The surgical procedure may involve use of plates, screws, and pins that are usually removed in the months after the operation.

The surgical procedures involved in reducing the hip are long and require an extended convalescence. Furthermore, there is a significant risk that what at first appears to be a successful technical result may turn into a stiff and painful joint (Fraser et al., 1980). Since such surgery is extremely demanding on the patient, family, and staff, it is not performed routinely on severely involved persons.

Occasionally, an orthopaedic surgeon may decide that it is necessary to perform an adductor muscle release even after a hip becomes dislocated. One of the first author's students with untreated

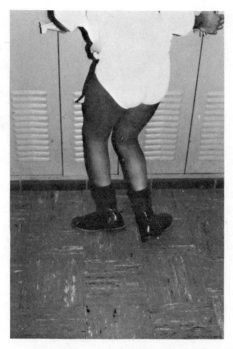

Figure 9.6. Postoperative appearance. This photograph of the student pictured in Figure 9.5 was taken 10 days after a surgical release of both hip adductor muscles. Note that she is now able to spread her legs enough to form a stable base for standing and can walk without her feet and legs crossing.

bilateral dislocated hips experienced a significant tightening of the adductor muscles during her early teens. This condition was causing her to lose the ability to walk (Figure 9.5) and to attend to her toileting needs since she could no longer separate her legs. The situation was brought to the attention of an orthopaedist who decided that surgery was needed to increase her hip range of motion. This facilitated improved perineal care and, at least temporarily, has helped her maintain her standing and walking skills. Her hospital stay was short—only a few days. She returned to school one week after surgery. Since she was not in a cast following surgery, standing and walking **(gait)** training were begun immediately upon her return to school (Figure 9.6). Although her hips remain dislocated, the surgical intervention produced a dramatic improvement in this student's ability to clean her perineum and take care of her menstrual flow. Her restored ability to bear weight to transfer in and out of a

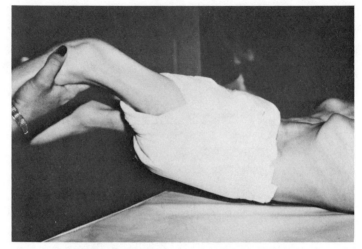

Figure 9.7. Hip extension deformity. Contractures have developed in the muscles that extend the upper legs. The therapist is able to flex this student's hips only a few degrees. Compare the limited hip flexion range of motion in this photograph with the normal range of motion in Figure 6.10.

wheelchair is a significant help to her care providers. The fact that she is able to walk with assistance following surgery is a bonus.

Readers are cautioned that not all persons will show such remarkable gains so quickly following surgery. In fact, many times it will take 6 months for a person to regain his or her preoperative level of physical function. This case is presented only to make the reader aware that, in certain cases, relatively simple procedures with appropriate physical therapy follow-up can make a great difference in an impaired person's ability to maintain good perineal hygiene.

Hip Extension Deformity

Hip extension deformities (Figure 9.7) fortunately are uncommon in neuromuscularly and severely involved persons (Bowen, MacEwen, & Mathews, 1981). This deformity is caused by contractures of the hip muscles that make the lower extremities extend. Persons with severe hip extension contractures eventually lose the ability to sit, and the hips may dislocate in a forward direction. When the deformity is mild, an affected individual should be positioned with hips flexed as much as possible. This may be accomplished by placing the person in a backlying (supine) position, with a bolster under the knees

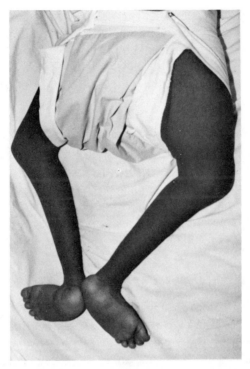

Figure 9.8. Hip abduction-flexion deformity. This deformity is sometimes called "frog legs" deformity because the legs are spread (abducted) and partly flexed, resembling a frog's hind legs.

to hold the hips and knees in a flexed position (see Figure 10.4). The person should spend as much time as comfortably possible in a chair during the day.

Surgical treatment of hip extension deformities consists of releasing the muscle contractures and is performed to maintain an individual's ability to sit and to relieve pain (Bowen et al., 1981).

Hip Abduction-Flexion Deformity

Hip abduction-flexion deformity causes an affected individual's legs to resemble frog legs (Figure 9.8). It may occur spontaneously, or arise as a complication of adductor release surgery (Fraser et al., 1980). Usually, it is not painful to the person, but it does interfere with positioning the individual in bed and in a sitting position. Sidelying is an excellent position for a person affected by a hip adduction-flexion deformity because the bed keeps the lower leg in position and gravity tends to pull the upper leg toward the midline. Adductor pads may be added to a wheelchair to keep the person's legs within the chair.

KNEE DEFORMITIES

Knee deformities are common among neuromuscularly and severely involved persons. Such deformities seldom present serious difficulty for those who are bedridden. However, knee deformities may interfere with standing balance for persons who are able to bear weight on their feet to transfer from wheelchair to bed and for those who can walk. Knee deformities may impose limitations on either of the two motions—flexion and extension—of which the joint is capable (Fraser et al., 1980).

Knee Flexion Deformity

Knee flexion deformity causes the lower leg to be held in a bent, contracted position. For a person who is bedridden, comfort is increased if he or she is placed in a sidelying or supine position. We recommend placing a bolster under the knees while the person is supine (see Figure 9.3). This prevents the legs from rotating to one side and, thus, keeps the pelvis and back in straighter alignment.

With persons who use a wheelchair, severe knee flexion will cause the back of the leg to wrap around the edge of the seat. This can be painful for the individual and makes it difficult for attendants to move him or her into and out of a chair.

When the deformity is mild, knee splints (Figure 9.9) can be used to keep the leg fairly straight for standing and for lying in a supine or sidelying position (Galka, Fraser, & Hensinger, 1980). Long leg braces (Figure 9.10), which were used at one time to keep the knee straight, are heavy, cumbersome, and difficult to fit. We do not recommend them for neuromuscularly involved or severely impaired persons.

Surgical Treatment Knee flexion deformity places strain on the knee cap **(patella)** and the tendon attachment to the shin bone **(tibia)**. This may cause an afflicted person to experience pain. Surgery (a soft tissue procedure) that involves lengthening the ham-

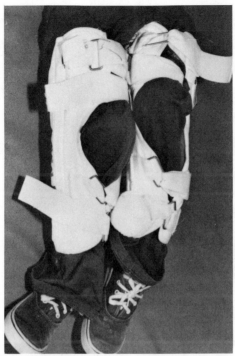

Figure 9.9. Knee splints. Knee splints are used to position slightly flexed knees in extension and as leg supports for short duration standing. Knee splints are available from Medipedic, Inc.

string muscles at the back of the thigh is seldom necessary for the wheelchair-bound individual, but may be considered for the ambulatory person to improve walking balance and relieve pain.

The hamstrings are the muscles behind the knee. They can be felt through the skin behind the knee. The hamstring muscles originate on the pelvis below the buttock and attach to the lower leg bone (tibia) below the knee. They help to extend the hip and bend the knee. Any change in their length can affect movement of both the hip and the knee.

In the early development of hamstring lengthening procedures, the tendons that attach the hamstrings to the tibia were transferred to the front of the kneecap to help in extension of the knee. Unfortunately, this resulted in gradual extension of the knee joint, which often became as much of a problem to the patient as the original knee

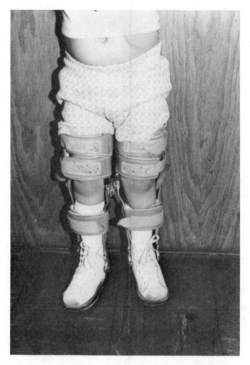

Figure 9.10. Long leg braces. In the past, braces such as these were commonly prescribed for neuromuscularly and severely involved persons. They are heavy, cumbersome, difficult to apply, and not helpful in long-term use in either preventing deformity or improving function.

flexion deformity. Presently, the surgical procedure is modified to lengthen the tendons of the hamstring muscles. In moderately involved patients, many surgeons leave one or more tendons intact.

Patients usually are kept in a cast following a hamstring lengthening procedure until the tendons heal—approximately 6 weeks. After cast removal, the patient is placed on a range of motion exercise program prescribed by a physical therapist. The effect of a hamstring lengthening procedure will not be fully realized for 6 months or more, when the other tissues about the joint have stretched out.

Knee Extension Deformity

Less commonly, an impaired individual may develop complete extension of one or both knees. This is especially likely to occur

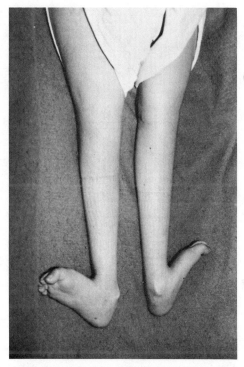

Figure 9.11. Knee extension deformity. This student's knees have been held in extension for many years due to spasticity of the muscle group on the front of the thigh (quadriceps). Her legs are so deformed that it is difficult to locate her knee cap (patella). In addition, her feet show a calcaneus deformity.

among persons whose abnormal muscle tone causes their legs to be held in a straight position (Figure 9.11). Sometimes, it can be a result of surgical overlengthening of a knee flexion contracture. Knee extension deformity may cause ambulatory individuals to lose the ability to walk. Wheelchair-bound persons should use elevating leg rests to support their legs (see Chapter 13).

Usually, persons with this kind of deformity will receive a continuing program of physical therapy. The goal of such a program is to maintain or increase joint flexion though positioning and exercise.

Surgical Treatment Surgery to correct a knee extension deformity usually consists of lengthening the **quadriceps** muscles. The quadriceps is the big muscle group on the front of the thigh that helps

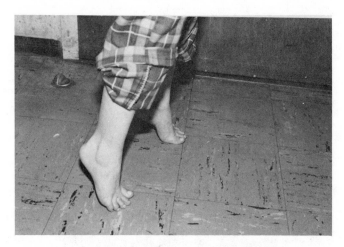

Figure 9.12. Equinus deformity. Tight heel cords cause this student to walk on his toes. Muscle and tendon tightness prevent his heels from touching the floor.

flex the hip and extend the knee. The postoperative period is similar to that for hamstring lengthening.

FOOT DEFORMITIES

Foot deformities are found frequently among neuromuscularly and severely involved persons, caused by unbalanced pull of muscles on the ankle and foot joints. There are four basic types of foot deformity corresponding to normal foot motions—down (**equinus**), up (**calcaneus**), in (**inversion**), and out (**eversion**). In addition, the forefoot may point in (varus) or out (valgus). In the following paragraphs, these deformities are described in more detail, after which treatments involving use of special shoes and braces and/or surgical correction are discussed.

Equinus Deformity

The most common foot deformity experienced by neuromuscularly and severely involved persons causes the heel to pull upward and the forefoot to point down, much like the position of a horse's hoof. In fact, the deformity's name, *equinus*, is derived from the Latin word *equino* meaning "of or like a horse." Equinus is caused by tightening of the **heel cord** located at the back of the ankle or by weakness of the

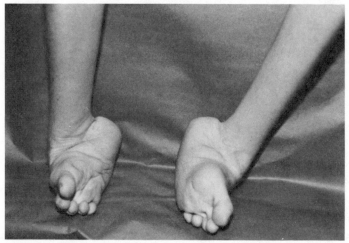

Figure 9.13. Inverted feet. These feet are severely deformed and fixed in an extreme inverted position.

muscles that **dorsiflex** the foot. Ambulatory persons with equinus deformity walk on their toes, with their heels off the floor (Figure 9.12).

Calcaneus Deformity

Calcaneus, the opposite deformity of equinus, occurs when the heel cord is too long or weak, and opposing muscles that flex the foot, pulling the forefoot upward, are too strong (see Figure 9.11). This deformity is found infrequently among neuromuscularly and severely involved persons (with the exception of persons with myelomeningocele spina bifida), which is fortunate because the deformity interferes with the individual's wearing shoes and bearing weight on the foot (Keats, 1970).

Inversion-Eversion Deformities

In combination with an equinus deformity, or separately, the inner (medial) side of a person's foot may pull upward (inversion) causing the person to walk on the outer edge of the foot (Figure 9.13). The opposite may also occur, creating a condition in which the outer (lateral) side of the foot pulls upward (eversion) causing the person to

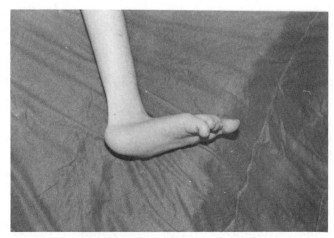

Figure 9.14. Everted foot. Persons with eversion deformity walk on the inner edge of the foot.

walk on the inner edge of the foot (sometimes called pronated or flat foot) (Figure 9.14).

Varus-Valgus Foot Deformities

Varus and valgus posture of the feet is used to describe the angulation created by abnormal muscle pull on the forefoot. A varus position

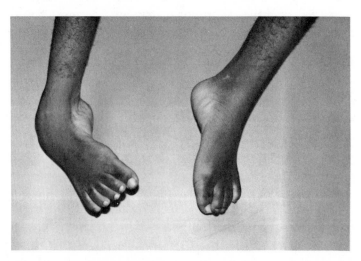

Figure 9.15. Varus deformities of the feet. Varus deformity of the feet can be recognized by the inward angulation of one or both forefeet.

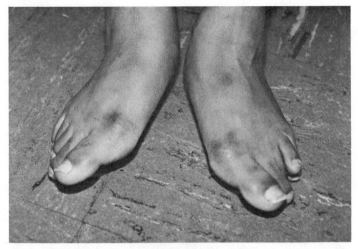

Figure 9.16. Valgus deformities of the feet. In the case of a valgus deformity, one or both forefeet angle out.

occurs when the forefoot curves inward (Figure 9.15). A valgus foot position occurs when one or both forefeet point outward away from each other (Figure 9.16).

Combination Foot Deformities

Combined foot deformities occur quite commonly in neuromuscularly and severely involved persons—equinovarus and equinovalgus. The equinovarus foot deformity (Figure 9.17) is caused by a tight heel cord, coupled with tightness of the posterior tibialis tendon and other structures in the medial side of the foot, making the forefoot turn inward and the individual walk up on the toes. In the equinovalgus deformity, the heel cord is tight, and there are tight structures in the lateral side of the foot producing a severe flat foot. This combination causes the forefoot to turn outward and the heel to be drawn upward. Thus, the foot appears to "break" at the midfoot (Figure 9.18). Equinovalgus deformity is often referred to as "rocker bottom foot."

Clawing of Toes

Clawing of the toes (Figure 9.19) may occur in conjunction with other foot deformities or in isolation. Toe clawing is usually triggered by a reflex action causing the toes to flex when pressure is applied to

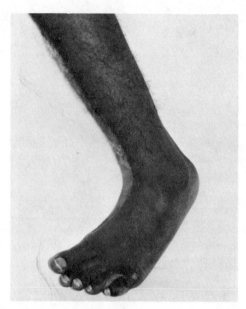

Figure 9.17. Equinovarus foot deformity. This deformity combines a tight heel cord with inward angulation of the forefoot.

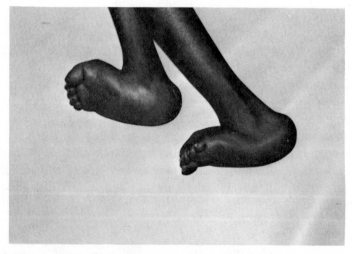

Figure 9.18. Equinovalgus foot deformity. This deformity is often called "rocker bottom foot."

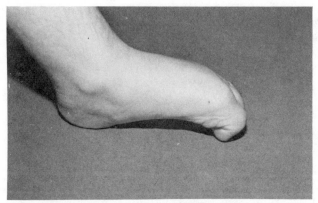

Figure 9.19. Clawing of toes. Clawing of the toes usually is caused by a reflex action that is abnormal if it occurs after about 9 months of age. Abnormal retention of this reflex may interfere with a child's learning to walk and eventually may lead to a fixed deformity.

the ball of the foot (Wilson, 1977). This reflex, called the **plantar grasp reflex,** occurs in normal infants for about the first 9 months of life and then integrates (disappears) into the central nervous system. In children with developmental and neuromuscular disabilities, the plantar grasp reflex may remain indefinitely (Effgen, 1982). This may eventually lead to a fixed deformity. When this occurs, surgical intervention may be necessary.

Treatment of Foot Deformities

Much like hip deformities, foot problems are so common among neuromuscularly and severely involved persons that they should be anticipated and attempts made to prevent deformity (Fraser et al., 1980). The goal of a prevention program is to keep the feet flexible enough to fit into shoes and remain flat to the floor **(plantigrade position).**

Shoes and Braces For very young handicapped children, a hightop orthopedic shoe with a hard sole (Figure 9.20) is recommended to hold the foot in proper position as it grows. Shoes should be carefully fitted by a trained specialist **(pedorthist)** and be worn as much as possible during the child's waking hours. Orthopedic shoes are designed to fit closely to the foot. Therefore, individuals who use them should wear thin, well-fitting socks to avoid pressure areas and

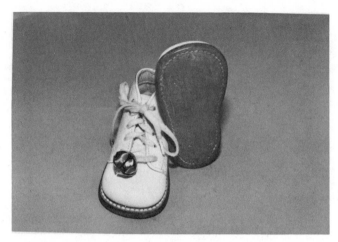

Figure 9.20. Hightop orthopedic shoes. This type of shoe is recommended for neuromuscularly and severely involved young children to hold the foot in proper position as it grows.

skin problems caused by sock wrinkles. The close fit also means that foot growth must be monitored carefully.

With development of spasticity, a child's heel cord may become tight. At this point, a short leg brace (Figure 9.21), attached to a hightop shoe, may be used to provide extra stability for the foot. However, long-term bracing generally is not very satisfactory for neurologically or severely involved persons, since most are unable to apply and care for their own braces (Fraser et al., 1980). In many cases, an operation to lengthen the **Achilles tendon** is preferable to bracing if the heel cord tightness cannot be controlled with simple measures.

In some instances, use of an ankle-foot orthosis shoe insert (Figure 9.22) may help to hold a foot in an acceptable position. Such orthoses (often called AFOs) are frequently prescribed for neuro-muscularly involved persons who have tight heel cords or who need foot stability. However, we do not recommend ankle-foot orthoses for severely impaired individuals because of danger that their skin may be unable to tolerate such a firm support. Furthermore, the ankle-foot orthosis is not effective in changing the foot or preventing deformity. It should also be noted that the ankle-foot orthosis is expensive and difficult to fit since it must conform exactly to the foot,

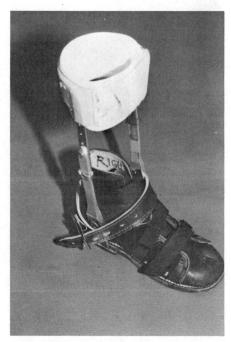

Figure 9.21. Short leg brace. The brace in this photograph consists of a calf band and two metal uprights attached to a hightop orthopedic shoe. Note that both the calf band and the shoe have Velcro closures for ease in applying the brace. If a strap is attached to a short leg brace, it should be buckled outside of the metal upright in order to hold the ankle in a straight position. It is a good idea to mark each student's shoes with his or her name and "right" or "left" to eliminate brace mix up and confusion about application to the correct foot.

and that these orthoses tend to be lost easily. For higher functioning children capable of self-care, AFOs may be used more successfully.

Care providers often complain of the struggle and time involved in placing orthopedic shoes and braces on severely impaired individuals. To simplify this process, ask that shoes be designed with a tongue extending all the way to the toe, and specify Velcro closures instead of laces (see Figure 9.21). These simple modifications cut the time required to put on braces considerably; in one case, the time needed was decreased from 15 minutes to less than 1 minute.

Toe clawing is troublesome because it makes shoe application difficult. For mild cases, it is helpful to have a shoe built up in the toe

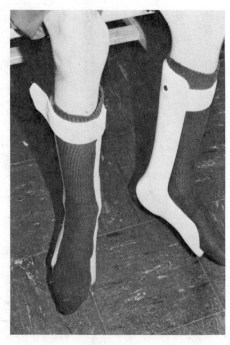

Figure 9.22. Ankle-foot orthosis (AFO). The AFO is molded to a person's foot. It is used much like the short leg brace to hold the foot in a corrected or more acceptable position. The AFO is worn inside a regular type shoe such as a tennis shoe.

area (toe crest) to take pressure off the ball of the foot (Figure 9.23) (Provost, 1982). In addition, a clear plastic insert may be placed over the toe area of the shoe so that the position of the toes may be monitored (Figure 9.24). In severe cases, the toe portion of the shoe may be removed (Figure 9.25). This eliminates pressure over the top of the toes and thus prevents skin breakdown. This modification also makes applying shoes much easier.

Shoes should be worn by all ambulatory and wheelchair-bound persons. Proper shoes improve balance and decrease potential for foot pain in individuals who have the ability to walk or stand. They also aid wheelchair-bound persons who often find it uncomfortable to rest bare or sock-clad feet on a metal footrest. Shoes also provide comfort, safeguard from injury, and protect against exposure to cold weather. Even severely deformed feet (see Figure 9.13) can and should be placed in tennis shoes (Figure 9.26). Bedridden persons, of

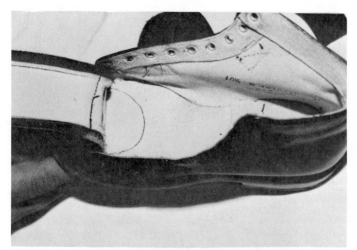

Figure 9.23. Toe crest. The toe portion of the sole (marked with pen) is padded to place most weight on the toes instead of the ball of the foot.

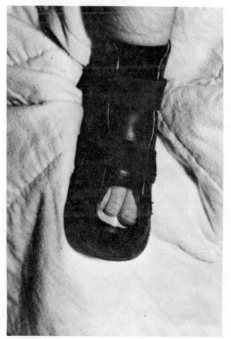

Figure 9.24. Plastic insert over toe area. This customized feature allows therapists and care providers to check the position of the toes.

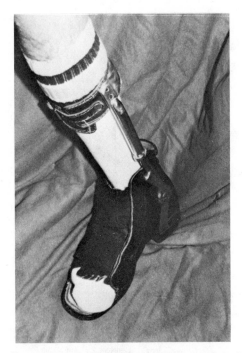

Figure 9.25. Shoe with toe portion removed. The top portion of the shoe's toe area is cut away to prevent pressure and skin breakdown on the top of the toes.

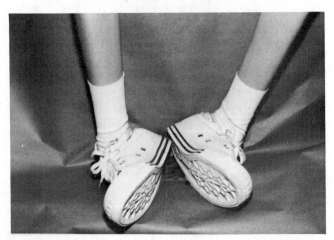

Figure 9.26. Severely deformed feet in tennis shoes. The deformed feet pictured in Figure 9.13 are placed in tennis shoes, which offer protection and conceal the severity of the deformity.

course, do not need shoes. Heavy socks that provide warmth are appropriate foot wear. They also reduce friction and the likelihood of heelsores.

Surgical Treatment of Foot Deformities In the case of neurologically involved individuals, surgical correction of foot deformities is normally performed to improve function. When dealing with severely impaired persons, surgery is employed most often to allow wearing of shoes and to improve appearance.

When the deformity is mild, soft tissue procedures, such as tendon lengthening or release, are effective in obtaining a normal foot position (Fraser et al., 1980). An example of a commonly performed soft tissue surgical procedure is a heel cord lengthening. The heel cord is just underneath the skin behind the ankle. An incision is made on the inner aspect and a little above the ankle (Figure 9.27). Care is taken not to put the scar directly on the posterior aspect over the heel cord since the scar could be susceptible to irritation caused by the heel rubbing on the back of the shoe.

There are a variety of ways to lengthen the heel cord, all of which are satisfactory. A popular method is described as a Z-lengthening, which involves cutting halfway through the tendon up high on the heel cord and halfway through the tendon down below on the opposite side. The two ends or tails are then sutured together.

The mechanism of lengthening is not too important. The key to the surgery is avoiding overlengthening of the heel cord. After surgery, if the foot goes up markedly into a flexed position (dorsiflexion), this can be as much a problem for the patient as the equinous was before surgery. Some surgeons recommend lengthening the heel cord about 10 to 15 degrees beyond the neutral position (indicated as 0 degrees in Figures 6.14 and 6.15) to avoid overlengthening of the heel cord. For severely impaired persons, we prefer the ankle to be held in a neutral position in the cast so there won't be any tension on the suture line.

At the time of surgery, the doctor may decide to lengthen other tendons in order to correct combined foot deformities. For example, if the tendons of the muscles that flex the toes are tight, the toes may curl when the foot is placed in a plantigrade or dorsiflexed position. A simple lengthening of the toe flexor tendons may be considered at the same time as the heel cord lengthening.

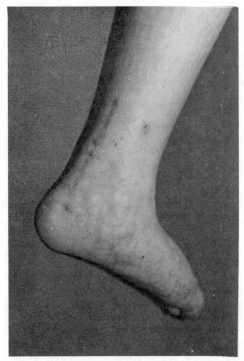

Figure 9.27. Heel cord surgical scar. This photograph of a student's heel cord surgical scar was taken the day after his casts were removed. Note that the scar occurs just medial to the back of the ankle. The incision is not made directly at the back of the ankle to protect the scar tissue from pressure and irritation created by the back of a shoe.

Following surgery, short leg casts (Figure 9.28) are applied and usually worn for about 6 weeks. Some surgeons prefer to use casts that extend over the knee. This can present a problem for severely handicapped persons, however, because it can lead to knee stiffness and skin breakdown. Consequently, applying a short leg cast may be more appropriate. If the patient is ambulatory, using a walking cast is often advisable to encourage the patient to bear weight on the feet so that strength is maintained in the quadriceps muscles.

It should be noted that after a short leg cast is removed, the muscles will be quite a bit weaker than they were before surgery, and the patient will need an exercise program prescribed and supervised by a physical therapist. If the person had been using short leg braces before the surgery, use of the braces is typically resumed after the

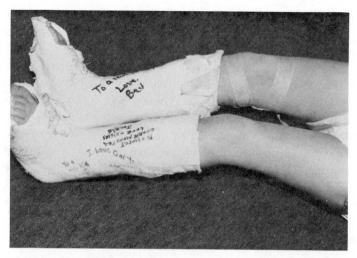

Figure 9.28. Short leg casts. This student had both heel cords lengthened at the same time. He wore casts for about 6 weeks after surgery and attended school during that time. He started standing on his feet about 4 weeks after surgery while he was still in the casts. Once the casts were removed, he used hightop shoes and short leg braces that had been ordered for him before the surgery.

casts are removed. The recovery period after surgery is only a month or two, and wearing the braces for a short period after casts are removed helps in building muscle strength.

If severe deformity develops, more complicated bony procedures are required to achieve a satisfactory position and stabilize the foot. In the older child or teenager with a stiff or rigid foot, a variation of the triple arthrodesis is usually the chosen method of treatment. This is a procedure that was used a great deal during the polio era to stabilize a deformed foot. It continues to be a popular, reliable procedure for neuromuscularly and severely impaired persons.

The triple arthrodesis consists of a fusion of the three joints of the hindfoot. A common confusion is that this procedure involves the ankle. It does not. It affects the joints immediately below the ankle and just in front of the ankle—the joints of the hindfoot. The bones are shaped so that they fit well and the foot is in a neutral position. This surgery may involve internal fixation of the bones with pins or staples until the fusion heals (in about 3 months' time). A long leg cast is applied for the first 6 weeks following surgery, and then a short leg cast is used for the last 6 weeks. In severely impaired persons, internal fixation is used more frequently than with other patients so that casting can be limited to a short leg cast for the entire 12 weeks of recuperation.

Some children will need foot stabilization at a relatively young age: 5–10 years. In such cases, an interim procedure is often suggested, called a Grice procedure. There are several technical variations of the Grice procedure that are not germane to this discussion. The basic principle of the Grice procedure, however, involves construction of a bony block between two major bones of the hindfoot (the **talus** and **os calcis**) to hold them in their normal positions relative to each other. This stabilization is done outside of the joint, and therefore is called an extra-articular arthrodesis. The Grice procedure allows the bones to continue to grow while they are held in the corrected position.

CONCLUSION

This discussion of lower extremity deformities is intended only to give the reader a basis for understanding how deformities occur and their influence on body posture and movement. This chapter can only serve as an introduction to a very complex subject. It takes many years of training and experience for orthopaedists and therapists to be qualified to analyze and treat persons with impairments such as those discussed in these pages.

REFERENCES

Bleck, E.E. Musculoskeletal examination of the child with cerebral palsy. *Developmental Medicine and Child Neurology*, 1979a, *23*, 23–39.

Bleck, E.E. *Orthopaedic management of cerebral palsy. Saunders Monographs in Clinical Orthopaedics*, Vol. 2. Philadelphia: W.B. Saunders Co. 1979b.

Bowen, J.R., MacEwen, G.D., & Mathews, P.A. Treatment of extension contractures of the hip in cerebral palsy. *Developmental Medicine and Child Neurology*, 1981, *23*, 23–29.

Effgen, S.K. Integration of the plantar grasp reflex as an indicator of ambulation potential in developmentally disabled infants. *Physical Therapy*, 1982, *62*(4), 433–435.

Fraser, B.F., Galka, G., & Hensinger, R.N. *Gross motor management of severely multiply impaired students, Vol. I: Evaluation guide*. Baltimore: University Park Press, 1980.

Galka, G., Fraser, B.A., & Hensinger, R.N. *Gross motor management of severely multiply impaired students, Vol. II: Curriculum model.* Baltimore: University Park Press, 1980.

Keats, S. *Operative orthopedics in cerebral Palsy.* Springfield, IL: Charles C Thomas, 1970.

Provost, B. PT practice tips. *Clinical Management in Physical Therapy,* 1982; 2, 1–4.

Samilson, R.L., Tsov, P., Aamoth, G., & Green, W.M. Dislocation and subluxation of the hip in cerebral palsy. Pathogenesis, natural history, and management. *Journal of Bone and Joint Surgery,* 1972, *54,* 863–873.

Wilson, J. A developmental reflex test. In: S.G. Volpe (ed.), *Volpe assessment battery for the atypical child.* Toronto: National Institute of Mental Retardation, 1977.

Postural Irregularities and Abnormal Balance Reactions

10

Irregular posture prevents coordinated body movement, interferes with development of gross motor skills (such as rolling, sitting, standing, and walking), and may lead to deformity. In severely impaired persons, irregular body posture is caused by abnormal muscle tone, abnormal **reflex** activity, or a combination of these factors. It is important that care providers recognize irregular posture and understand why it occurs so that they will handle impaired persons effectively and position them correctly.

This chapter first discusses abnormal muscle tone and then examines abnormal reflexes that affect posture. Subsequently, certain balance reactions, which, if absent, involve serious handling implications, are considered.

ABNORMAL MUSCLE TONE

Most adolescents and adults with brain damage suffer from the effects of too much muscle tone (hypertonia) or a permanent increase

157

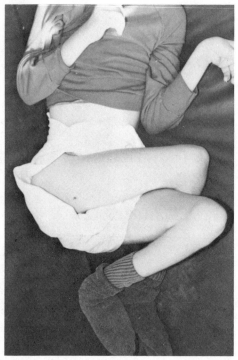

Figure 10.1. Crossed legs. The boy pictured lying on his side with legs crossed is 19 years old. The adductor muscles of both hips have been tight for many years. In his childhood, the muscle tightness caused his legs to draw together. During a growth spurt in his early teens, the muscle tightness increased further, causing him to cross his legs. At present, the position of his legs shown in this photograph is the only one that he can tolerate. This problem might have been prevented if a surgical release of the tight hip muscles had been done before contractures became severe.

in muscle tone (spasticity) (Bleck, 1979b). An example of hypertonia that affects the entire body is **extensor thrust** (discussed below). Spasticity is commonly found in the thigh muscles where it can cause the legs (hip adductor muscles) to pull together (Figure 10.1) (Bleck, 1979a). This results in persistent crossing of the legs, known as scissoring. The following paragraphs describe in detail the problems and care techniques associated with these two postural irregularities.

Extensor Thrust

Severely impaired persons may show a backward (extensor) thrust of the upper body and, sometimes, of the legs when they are in

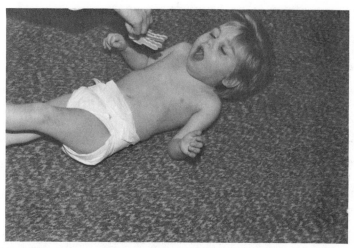

Figure 10.2. Extensor thrust prohibits sitting. This student is 3 years old. He is alert, sees the keys, and wants to sit up and touch them. One can tell that he is putting forth great effort in his attempt to sit because he is bending his legs and head, and the strain causes him to open his mouth. Unfortunately, despite a total body effort, extensor thrust keeps him pinned to the floor.

reclining, sitting, and standing positions. Extensor thrust, unlike opisthotonos (see Chapter 7), occurs sporadically and may be controlled by positioning. Care providers can help to lessen the effects of extensor thrust by keeping the impaired person in a flexed position whenever practicable.

Backlying Positioning When in a backlying position, a person who experiences extensor thrust appears to be pinned to the floor by some invisible force. In fact, the extensor thrust may be so strong that the person is unable to lift his or her head (Figure 10.2) or roll over (Figure 10.3) (Wilson, 1977).

When such a person is resting in a backlying position, extensor thrust may be eased by placing a pillow under the shoulders, neck, and head, and by placing a bolster under the thighs, just above the knees (Figure 10.4). This will hold the head, torso, hips, and knees in flexion.

Sitting Position When in a sitting position, the hips of a person with extensor thrust will spring forward, appearing to launch the individual out of the seat (Figure 10.5) (Fraser, Galka, & Hensinger, 1980). Individuals with strong extensor thrust need to be

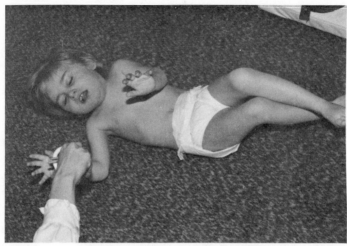

Figure 10.3. Extensor thrust inhibits rolling. The therapist has moved the keys to the student's right side to encourage him to roll over. Again, he is trying with all his strength to roll toward the keys, but cannot overcome the effects of extensor thrust.

held in their chair by a seat T-strap (Figure 10.6) placed between the legs and tied in back of the chair to help anchor the buttocks in the chair. A neck support may be added to the chair (Figure 10.7) to hold the head in a flexed position. (Be certain that the right kind of device is used and that it makes contact in the neck area. Placing pressure on the back of the head will trigger extensor thrust.) A lap tray will allow

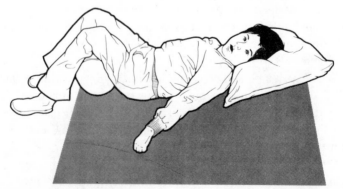

Figure 10.4. Backlying position for extensor thrust. The boy in this illustration is placed in a backlying position with a pillow under his head, neck, and shoulders, and a bolster under his thighs. This flexed position lessens the effects of extensor thrust.

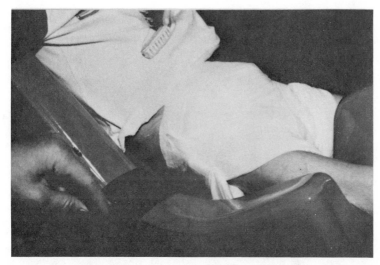

Figure 10.5. Extensor thrust causes sitting problems. This child's extensor thrust became severe by age 12, causing his body to be stiff and straight. Even when placed in a soft curved seat, his hips will not relax enough to allow his buttocks to touch the seat. As shown in this photograph, extensor thrust appears to launch him out of the seat.

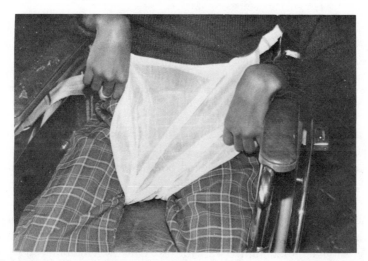

Figure 10.6. T-strap. When an impaired person with extensor thrust is able to sit in a standard wheelchair, a T-strap should be used to anchor the buttocks in the chair. The T-strap is placed between the legs and secured to the back of the wheelchair. It may be used in addition to a regular wheelchair seat belt. T-straps are available from T. J. Posey Company.

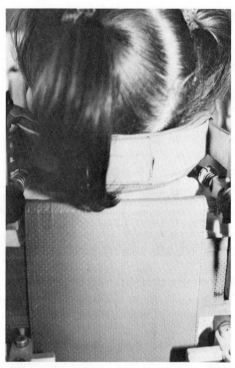

Figure 10.7. Neckrest used to control extensor thrust. Because this girl, age 9, has extensor thrust, she uses a neckrest instead of a headrest when sitting in her wheelchair. The neckrest provides adequate support for her head without touching the back of her skull, which would trigger extensor thrust. Supported in the manner shown, she has improved use of her hands when operating her communication board (see Figure 11.2).

the arms to rest in a forward position. The hips, knees, and ankles should be flexed to a right angle if possible. The object of positioning in a chair is to encourage a flexed body posture to counteract the backward pull of the extensor thrust.

Standing Position When a person with extensor thrust is standing, it looks as if someone were behind him or her pulling back on the shoulders. It is difficult for a person affected by extensor thrust to get enough momentum to walk forward or to even maintain enough balance to stand. The impaired person will need to hold onto an object such as a table or chair, placed in front of him or her, to be able to

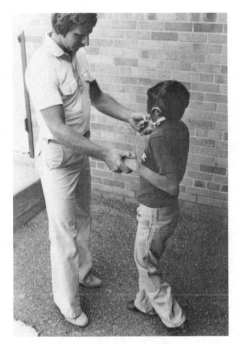

Figure 10.8. The teacher in this illustration stands to the front and side of this student with extensor thrust to direct his weight shifts during walking forward.

stand. To walk, he or she will need assistance: stay in front of the individual and hold onto a hand; move backward slowly as the individual steps forward, continuing to hold onto the person to help him or her maintain balance. This positioning will help keep the person's weight directed forward (Figure 10.8).

Scissoring

The majority of severely impaired persons experience spasticity of the hip adductor muscles. This limits the movement of the legs away from the midline and may cause the legs to cross (see Figure 10.1). Such a closed leg position, plus the constant pull of spastic adductor muscles, makes it difficult to separate the legs for a diaper change and for cleaning of the perineal area. Spastic muscle tightness may be reduced through relaxation techniques. To change the diaper of a person whose legs scissor, the following steps are suggested:

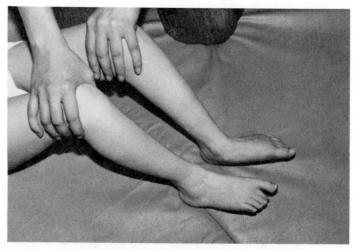

Figure 10.9. Relaxation before a diaper change. The helper places her hands on the impaired person's knees in order to gently roll the legs and hips from side to side. This slow rhythmical motion relaxes tight hip muscles. The helper then is able to separate the person's legs by gently spreading the knees.

Place the person in a backlying position.

Gently bend the knees and place your hands over the person's kneecaps.

Roll the legs and hips from side to side slowly and rhythmically (Figure 10.9), controlling the person's movements from the knees.

Gently separate the legs by pulling the knees apart once lessening of tension is evident in the thighs.

Proceed to change the diaper.

Do *not* try to separate scissoring legs (Figure 10.10) by pulling them apart while holding onto the ankles (Figure 10.11). This will only serve to increase the spasticity and make the legs close together more tightly. Instead, gently separate the legs while holding the knees in a slightly bent position (Figure 10.12). As mentioned in Chapter 9, bolsters or chair abductor pads may be used to separate the legs during rest in a backlying or sitting position.

ABNORMAL REFLEX ACTIVITY

A **postural reflex** is an involuntary reaction that changes the position of parts of the body. A detailed study of such reflexes is important to

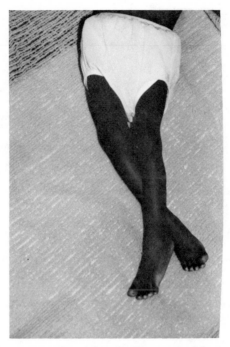

Figure 10.10. Scissoring legs. Hip adductor muscle tightness causes this boy's legs to be held in an extended position, with crossing at the ankles. This crossing action is called *scissoring* because the muscle tightness in the hips causes the legs to resemble the action of scissors.

doctors in establishing a diagnosis and predicting future progress (prognosis) in gross motor skills. Therapists test reflexes to help determine a child's developmental age and for use as a guide in planning a treatment or management program (Fraser et al., 1980). It is beyond the scope of this book to cover this complex subject in detail. However, care providers should be aware of the abnormal occurrence of two reflexes, the **asymmetrical tonic neck reflex (ATNR)** and the **Moro reflex,** which call for special precautions in handling affected persons.

Asymmetrical Tonic Neck Reflex

The asymmetrical tonic neck reflex is activated by turning the affected person's head to the side. This head movement causes the individual to assume a "fencing position": the arm toward which the face is turned extends, and the opposite arm flexes (Figure 10.13).

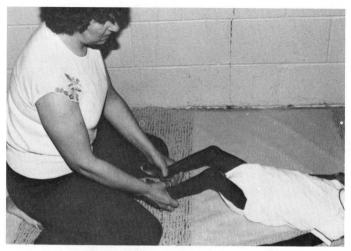

Figure 10.11. Incorrect separation of scissoring legs. The instructional aide shows that handling scissoring legs by the ankles is not an effective way of separating them. Tight adductor muscles will not allow the legs to be separated any further than shown when held by the ankles. The straight leg position places extra stress on the hip adductor muscles thereby adding to the spasticity.

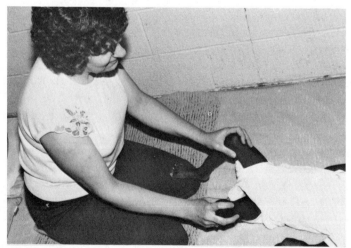

Figure 10.12. Correct separation of scissoring legs. Working with the same boy pictured in Figure 10.11, the instructor demonstrates the increased range of motion that can be achieved by using the correct technique—student's knees bent with instructional aide's hands on the knees and applying gentle pressure to spread the legs.

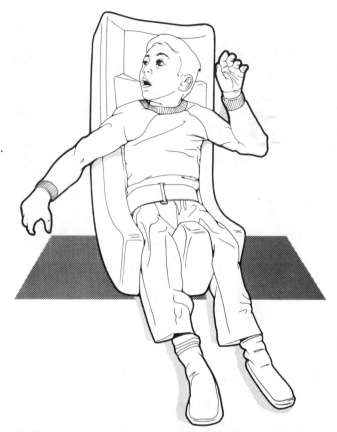

Figure 10.13. Asymmetrical tonic neck reflex. As shown in this illustration, the ATNR causes a student to assume a ''fencing'' position every time his head is turned.

This reflex may occur when the face is turned only toward one side, or it may occur when the face is turned to either side. If the reflex is particularly strong, it may cause a similar reaction to take place in the legs.

The ATNR may be present at birth in any infant, but it normally disappears (integrates) into the nervous system around 3 to 5 months of age (Wilson, 1977), as the child learns to bring his or her hands together in a midline position. In brain damaged children, however, the ATNR may persist past this stage of development and become abnormal (pathological). Therapy in young children is directed

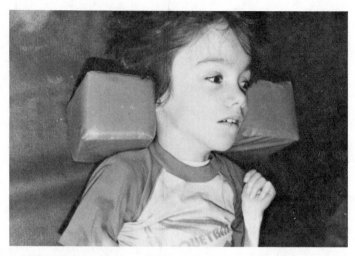

Figure 10.14. Supine headrest. This student uses a headrest while in a backlying position on the mat because he is unable to hold his head in a midline placement. His teacher places objects of interest directly above his face in order to keep his attention straight ahead and lessen the effects of the ATNR.

toward helping this reflex integrate. Such therapy usually includes positioning techniques. However, if ATNR is present in an adolescent or adult, we may presume that the reflex will not be integrated or overcome, and that we must accommodate its existence to the extent possible by handling and positioning so as to avoid triggering the abnormal reaction.

The ATNR is particularly troublesome because it prevents a person's hands from being brought together when the head is turned. Imagine how frustrating it must be for an individual whose arm flings out every time the head is turned. If a normal person were to assume such a "fencing position" while sitting, an unbalanced weight distribution would occur that would quickly become quite uncomfortable. In impaired persons, the asymmetrical posture caused by the ATNR can lead to deformities such as scoliosis and hip subluxation or dislocation.

Persistence of the ATNR makes walking unlikely (Capute, 1979). If the ATNR is present along with other abnormal reflexes, the likelihood of ambulation is still further reduced (Bleck, 1979b). Techniques to help the individual cope with the ATNR when reclin-

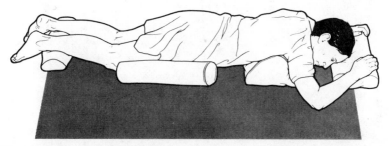

Figure 10.15. Prone positioning for ATNR. This illustration depicts a male student in a facelying position with a bolster under his chest and a towel roll under his forehead. This position ensures ample breathing space and helps hold his head in a midline alignment. A small roll under his ankles keeps pressure off his toes, while a bolster at his side offers further support to keep the hips in a straight position.

ing or sitting, however, can be implemented. For either activity, to inhibit this reflex, the head must be maintained in a centered (midline) position. If a person cannot maintain his or her head in this position while backlying, sandbags or headrests (Figure 10.14) may be placed beside either cheek. Objects of interest should be placed directly above the face to encourage holding the midline position. If the individual is in a facelying position, a bolster or wedge may be placed under the chest and a towel roll under the forehead (Figure 10.15). Arms should be positioned forward so the forearms rest on the mat. A sidelying position is excellent for any person with ATNR because the head is supported in a midline position by a pillow (Figure 10.16) (Galka, Fraser, & Hensinger, 1980). In a wheelchair, a person affected by ATNR persistence will need a headrest to hold the midline position. By keeping the head centered, the impaired person may be able to use both hands for an activity placed on a lap tray. When speaking to the individual, stand in front of the person with your face at his or her face level. Do not call to the person from the side. Doing so encourages turning the head, which will stimulate the unwanted reflex.

Moro Reflex

The Moro reflex is triggered by sudden removal of support while a person is being lowered from a sitting into a backlying position. It

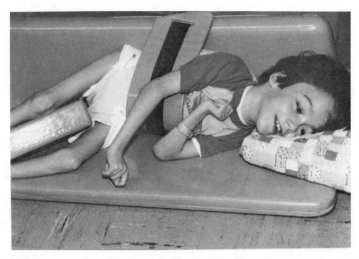

Figure 10.16. Sidelying positioning for ATNR. This student uses a sidelying positioner that lets him bring his arms together while his head is held in midline to decrease the effects of the ATNR. The positioner is available from J. A. Preston Corporation.

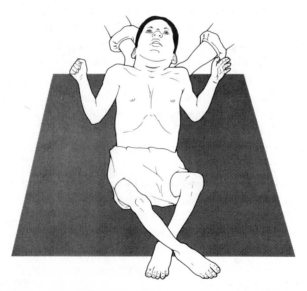

Figure 10.17. Moro Reflex. This illustration depicts a student's Moro reflex. When support for a sitting position was removed quickly, the boy flung his arms out away from his body, and his head dropped backward.

causes the arms to shoot away from the body (Figure 10.17). A Moro reflex interferes with obtaining head control and using the arms to help regain lost balance. Care providers should be certain to support the head and upper body when lowering an individual with this reflex from a sitting into a supine position. Care should also be taken when repositioning the back of an affected individual's wheelchair not to recline it quickly and thereby trigger this reaction.

BALANCE REACTIONS

Certain postural reactions are helpful to normal babies learning to sit and stand. In fact, once fully developed (at 6–18 months in normal children), these reactions remain throughout life (Wilson, 1977). Two such reactions are **protective extension,** which helps with

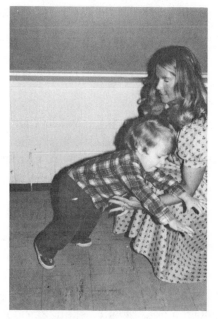

Figure 10.18. Protective extension reaction. A teacher pushes her student off balance to demonstrate his protective extension reaction. As shown in the photograph, when pushed, the student's arms automatically extend to block a fall and protect his head from damage. Once developed, this reaction normally lasts throughout life.

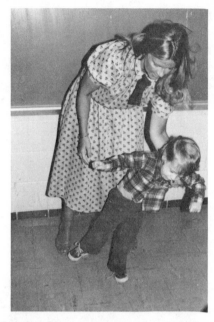

Figure 10.19. Negative sideways staggering reaction. If pushed sideways, the student would fall because his staggering reaction is not developed as yet.

sitting and standing balance, and **staggering reactions,** which are needed for standing and walking balance. Care providers need to know whether or not the persons they handle lack these reactions so that they are prepared to offer them adequate protection from a fall.

Protective Extension

The protective extension reaction is present if a person quickly extends both arms when pushed off balance from a sitting or standing position (Figure 10.18). This reaction is used to block a fall when pushed in a forward, backward, or sideways direction. The protective extension reaction is important because it helps to protect the face in case of a fall. If the reaction is absent, a person still may have the ability to maintain a nonsupported sitting position, but will not be able to counteract a loss of balance and protect his or her head from hitting the floor. Persons who have not developed this reaction should have support when sitting and should never be left in an unrestrained sitting position without supervision.

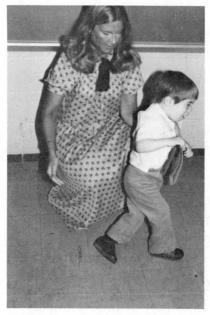

Figure 10.20. Positive sideways staggering reaction. This student is a bit upset about being pushed off balance to the side. As shown in the photograph, he maintains his balance by side stepping.

Staggering Reactions

Most severely impaired persons, even if they have the ability to stand or take a few steps with assistance, do *not* have the ability to cross-step when pushed sideways (Figures 10.19 and 10.20) or to counter a forward or backward loss of balance (Figures 10.21 and 10.22). Individuals who lack this balance mechanism (staggering reaction) should not stand without someone present to supervise. During standing or walking practice, a helmet should be worn as head protection in case of a fall.

CONCLUSION

This information on postural irregularities can provide only the most basic kind of overview for what is a very complex subject. Readers who are personally involved with the care of a severely impaired

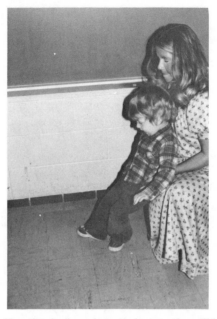

Figure 10.21. Negative backward staggering reaction. This photograph shows that the student is just beginning to develop a backward staggering reaction. Until such time as the reaction is fully developed, he is in danger of falling backward if balance is lost.

person are advised to discuss care requirements and handling techniques for that particular person with the attending therapist.

REFERENCES

Bleck, E.E. Musculoskeletal examination of the child with cerebral palsy. *Pediatric Annals,* 1979a, *8*(10), 31–37.

Bleck, E.E. *Orthopaedic management of cerebral palsy. Saunders Monographs in Clinical Orthopaedics, Vol. 2.* Philadelphia: W.B. Saunders Co., 1979b.

Capute, A.J. Identifying cerebral palsy in infancy through study of primitive reflex profiles. *Pediatric Annals,* 1979, *8*(10), 16–20.

Fraser, B.A., Galka, G., & Hensinger, R.N. *Gross motor management of severely multiply impaired students, Vol. 1: Evaluation guide.* Baltimore: University Park Press, 1980.

Galka, G., Fraser, B.A., & Hensinger, R.N. *Gross motor management of severely*

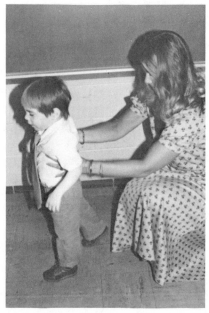

Figure 10.22. Positive backward staggering reaction. The student backsteps to maintain his balance when pushed. Therefore, we may assume that he can safely walk independently.

multiply impaired students, Vol. II: Curriculum model. Baltimore: University Park Press, 1980.

Wilson, J. A developmental reflex test. In: S.G. Volpe (ed.), *Assessment battery for the atypical child.* Toronto: National Institute of Mental Retardation, 1977.

Section III

TECHNIQUES
AND TIPS
FOR HELPING
THOSE WITH
SEVERE
IMPAIRMENTS

Communicating with Severely Impaired Persons

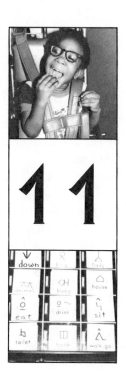

It is essential for care providers to gain at least a basic knowledge of communication techniques used by severely impaired persons before working with them. At first, this may seem to be a formidable task. However, most people quickly learn the nonverbal communication methods used by severely impaired individuals, become adept at understanding their special needs, and enjoy socializing with them.

The majority of severely impaired persons cannot speak. This does not necessarily mean that they do not understand what is said to them. Because it sometimes seems as if the mental abilities that severely impaired persons possess are held hostage by the physical imperfections of their bodies, it is difficult to know how much they do understand (**receptive language**). For this reason, it is best when speaking to a severely impaired person to:

Keep sentences short and simple.
Speak slowly, wait between thoughts, and watch for a response.
Give the person the benefit of the doubt; assume that he or she
  understands.

It is important to realize that the response you receive will not necessarily be verbal. It may be eye or hand movement; a change in bodily tension; or, perhaps, a laugh or a cry.

Because it is unclear how much is understood, be careful not to make unkind remarks in front of a severely impaired individual. In one situation, a visitor to a classroom was overheard commenting about a student's body odor. The student immediately became tense and anxious. In another incident, a teacher noticed that a severely impaired student laughed at subtle jokes, a sign of intelligence previously undetected in that student.

INDIRECT COMMUNICATION

Sometimes, it is possible to communicate in indirect ways with students who do not respond to spoken words. For instance, a child may be instructed to roll over by pushing on a shoulder to stimulate him or her into performing the desired movement. Or, placing a brightly colored object or favorite toy just out of reach may motivate a child to roll toward it. Teachers of severely impaired students often use this type of communication, sometimes called physical prompting, to help their students learn movement (gross motor) skills (Galka, Fraser, & Hensinger, 1980).

COMMUNICATION METHODS AND EQUIPMENT

Imagine how terribly frustrating it would be to understand what is said to you but not be able to respond. Many severely impaired individuals have receptive language but they are unable to speak, to write, or even to produce symbolic gestures (**gestural language**). The effort that they must make to communicate can seem overwhelming. But, with the help of a speech-language pathologist, some severely impaired persons may learn to use communication boards, such as a picture board (Figure 11.1), a word symbol board (Figure 11.2), or a "talking machine" (Figure 11.3), to express their needs and thoughts (Silverman, 1980). Methods of indicating a response may be as simple as looking at an object (eye pointing), using aids such as a head pointer (Figure 11.4) or a light pointer (Figure 11.5), or operating electronic devices by hand, foot, or head controls. Other

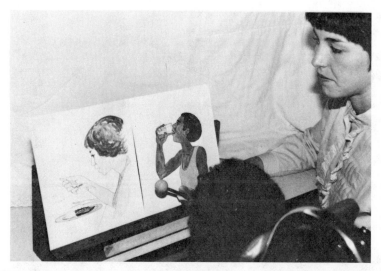

Figure 11.1. Picture board. This student uses a xylophone stick attached to a palmar band to point to a picture on the board. The pointer was designed for him by an occupational therapist. Notice that the pictures represent two basic needs—drinking and eating. This arrangment of pictures enables him to indicate to his speech-language pathologist whether he is thirsty or hungry. The pictures are large because his hand and arm coordination is poor and he would have difficulty pointing to a small sized picture.

individuals who have controlled use of their arms and hands may learn a sign (gestural) method of communication (Figure 11.6).

While use of a communication board and gestures (**augmentative communication systems**) enhances a nonspeaking person's ability to communicate, readers should be aware that the process is very slow. It is important that the impaired individual not sense any impatience on the part of the listener. Nonverbal communication is hard work for the severely impaired person, and discouragement can easily prevent the effort from being made.

Readers interested in learning about the characteristics, advantages, and limitations of various types of augmentative communication systems may want to consider Franklin H. Silverman's book, *Communication for the Speechless* (Silverman, 1980).

Engineers and speech-language pathologists are working to expand and improve communication aids and techniques. The rapid rate of new developments in this area make it difficult to present the

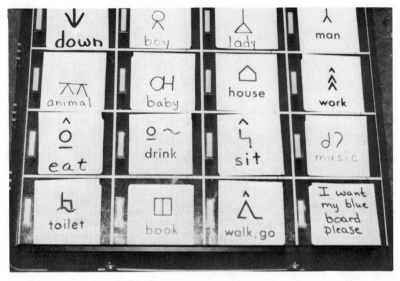

Figure 11.2. Word symbol board. This word symbol board is a more advanced type of communication system than the picture board in Figure 11.1 because symbols are used instead of pictures. Each symbol represents a word, such as house and book. As many as 16 symbols may appear on this board. The speech-language pathologist arranged these symbols for a particular student on a Zygo Communication Board available from Everest and Jennings. The student uses a touch-sensitive switch control to activate signal lights located by each square to indicate the symbol she desires.

most current information in a book. However, an excellent newsletter, *Communication Outlook,* published by the Artificial Language Laboratory, Computer Science Department, Michigan State University, East Lansing, Michigan 48824, keeps its readers posted on new equipment and training techniques.

SCHOOL SPEECH-LANGUAGE THERAPY

A visitor to a school for physically and mentally handicapped students may find it interesting to watch a speech-language pathologist assess a student's language abilities, select the most appropriate means of communication, and assist the student in developing language skills. Speech-language pathologists often work with school physical and occupational therapists when deciding upon a com-

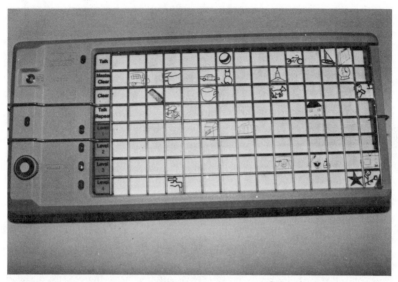

Figure 11.3. "Talking machine." This battery-operated Votrax Handivoice Communication Board is preprogrammed with 373 words and 16 short phrases. The speech-language pathologist may use graphics, symbols, or written language overlays with the board. After the student touches the display area, the Handivoice pronounces the indicated word or phrase. Sophisticated communication systems like the Handivoice are expensive and, unfortunately, most are not funded by a patient's health insurance. Such "talking machines" make excellent gifts for a special education program (for example, from an interested local civic organization), since they can be used by more than one student. Handivoice is available from Phonic Ear Ltd.

munication system. For example, the physical therapist may determine the seating position that will allow the impaired person to use hand, foot, or head controls most effectively. (In Chapters 10 and 12, how therapeutic positioning helps to diminish abnormal reflexes that affect posture and lessen the person's ability to control arm, leg, or head movements is discussed.) The occupational therapist may be called upon to make a special hand pointer for a student who cannot grasp properly. If a student shows potential toward developing verbal skills, the occupational therapist may prescribe lip and tongue exercises that help prepare mouth muscles for speaking (Silverman, 1980). The speech-language pathologist, in return, offers valuable advice to the physical and occupational therapist on how to communicate with individual students.

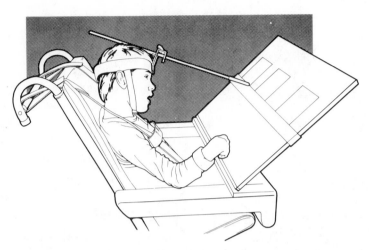

Figure 11.4. Head pointer. The student in this illustration is using a pointer attached to a headband to indicate his choice of pictures on the board. He does not have controlled use of his hands, but does have sufficient head control to use the head pointer. A pointing device similar to the one illustrated is available from Fred Sammons, Inc.

Because nonverbal methods are not perceived as the ''normal'' way to communicate, motivating students to use special devices can be difficult. Students may be very sensitive to the fact that they are ''different.'' For example, one of the first author's students was

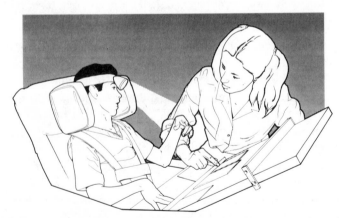

Figure 11.5. Light pointer. A lighted head pointer also may be used by students who lack hand control but who do have fair head control. Light pointers may be purchased from Brookstone Co.

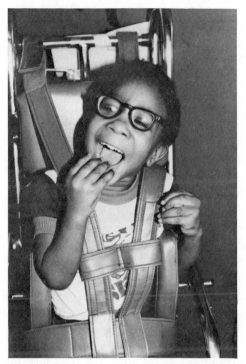

Figure 11.6. Gestural communication. This student says that he is hungry!

equipped with a system that was perfect for her physical needs, but after a couple of weeks she stopped using it. Instead, she kept attempting to talk, although the only sound she could make was "ah." Her teacher and speech-language pathologist realized that she did not like being different from the other students in her classroom who were verbal. To help her accept reality, both her parents and school staff began talking to her about her handicaps, explaining to her that she would never be able to talk no matter how hard she tried, but that she could communicate her needs and feelings by using her communication system. Such directness is hard for any of us, but it can be the best therapeutic approach in some situations. Happily this student understood and accepted her situation and now she is communicating effectively using her nonverbal system.

Parents and care providers can be of invaluable help in assisting severely impaired children to develop language skills. Although one should always seek and follow the advice of the attending speech-language pathologist when dealing with an individual student, some general guidelines may be helpful. The following suggestions (P. Cunningham, 1982, personal communication) should be helpful for anyone dealing with a nonverbal person:

1. *Begin early.* Start talking to the child as soon as he or she becomes aware of people and things in the environment. Talk about objects that are used daily, such as a cup, spoon, and brush. Name the body parts and items of clothing. It is very important to talk to a nonverbal child in order to help him or her develop a receptive vocabulary. Most of a physically impaired child's information is obtained through the auditory sense because movement limitations do not allow him or her to explore and learn by touching.

2. *Offer choices.* To establish a stimulating environment that will promote the desire to communicate, create situations where the student is allowed to make choices. At meal time, hold up two food items and let the student choose one. Encourage the student to select recreational activities by asking whether he or she would, for example, like to listen to music or go for a walk. It is best to avoid *yes* and *no* questions, at least initially. Normally children do not use "yes" and "no" reliably until they are between 2 and 3 years of age, so it is inadvisable to expect a *yes/no* response from a severely impaired student who may be functioning at a 1- or 2-year developmental age level.

3. *Avoid abstract concepts.* Avoid the use of symbols that require abstract thinking. For instance, if a student experiences pain after prolonged sitting, he or she needs a means to communicate the desire to get down on the mat. Therefore, a symbol for mat should be provided, not a symbol for pain. The student may know what pain means, but may not associate it with solving his or her problem.

Readers interested in obtaining information about the profession of speech-language pathology may contact the American Speech-Language-Hearing Association at 10801 Rockville Pike, Rockville, Maryland 20852. The Association's toll free phone number is 1-800-638-6868.

CONCLUSION

Nonverbal severely impaired persons require special systems to communicate basic needs and desires. Team effort by parents, care providers, and the speech-language pathologist is needed if such communication is to be effective. It is extremely rewarding for all concerned to see a nonverbal person communicate for the first time and to know that they played a part in this process.

REFERENCES

Galka, G., Fraser, B.A., & Hensinger, R.N. *Gross motor management of severely multiply impaired students, Vol. I: Evaluation guide*. Baltimore: University Park Press, 1980.

Silverman, P.H. *Communication for the speechless*. Englwood Cliffs, NJ: Prentice-Hall, 1980.

Handling Severely Impaired Persons with Abnormal Body Posture

12

This chapter discusses **body mechanics** techniques and handling suggestions that can make lifting impaired persons easier for care providers and more comfortable for the individual. The material presented is geared toward deformed adolescents and adults. Readers interested in techniques appropriate for infants and young cerebral palsied children are encouraged to consider Nancie Finnie's book, *Handling the Young Cerebral Palsied Child at Home* (Finnie, 1975).

BODY MECHANICS

Use of correct and efficient body movements, known as body mechanics, helps prevent pulled muscles, strained backs, and other problems related to improper posture. Learn and practice good body mechanics! When working with severely impaired persons, care providers and parents should think of themselves as well as the handicapped individual. Let's review a few ways to prevent back strain and make the job of lifting easier:

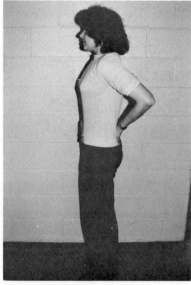

Figure 12.1. Setting the pelvis. This special education teacher shows the correct way to "set" the pelvis prior to lifting. She tightens both abdominal and buttock muscles while taking a deep breath. This simple exercise helps strengthen the muscles and protects the back against strain.

1. Learn to "set" the pelvis before lifting. This is done by tightening abdominal muscles and buttocks at the same time (Figures 12.1 and 12.2). Taking a deep breath as these muscles are tightened will help one learn to "set" the pelvis. This simple exercise prepares the body for strenuous lifting.

2. Bend from the knees (Figure 12.3), not from the waist (Figure 12.4). If an impaired person is lying on a floor mat, the lifter kneels on one knee beside the person and lifts by using the strong thigh muscles (Figure 12.5). The low back should be kept as vertical as possible during the lift.

3. Pull, don't push, when moving an impaired person in bed. Stand beside the bed, and pull the person toward the edge. If the impaired person is on a floor mat, kneel on the mat and pull him or her across the mat. (It is much easier to pull a heavy object toward oneself than to push that object away.)

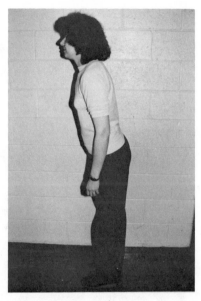

Figure 12.2. Relaxed posture. This photograph demonstrates poor or relaxed standing posture. If the teacher were to lift a heavy object with her low back curved in this way, she would place extra strain on her spinal muscles.

4. Carry an impaired person close to the body (Figure 12.6). Holding a person away from the body places extra strain on the back (Figure 12.7).

For a more detailed study of body mechanics, readers might refer to Helen Millen's book, *Body Mechanics and Safe Transfer Techniques* (Millen, 1974).

LIFTING METHODS

Most severely impaired persons are unable to understand or physically assist in the transfer process. Transfer techniques used most frequently in a special education setting involve moving a student from a floor mat to a wheelchair and vice versa. Some small students can be lifted safely by one person. However, most require a two-person lift. In some cases, three people will be needed to transfer a

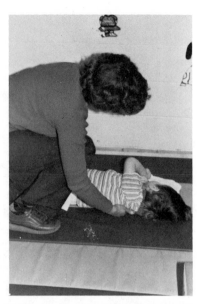

Figure 12.3. Correct bending. By bending from her knees, the teacher takes strain off her back and uses her thigh muscles to assist with lifting.

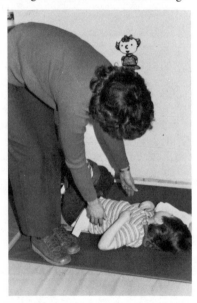

Figure 12.4. Incorrect bending. Because this teacher bends from her waist instead of her knees, she places extra stress on her back when picking up the child.

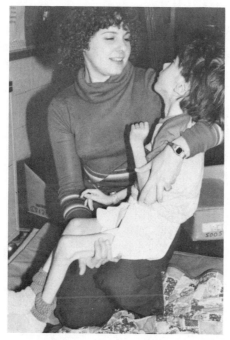

Figure 12.5. Lifting student from a mat. This teacher demonstrates the correct method for lifting her student, from a floor mat. Notice that she is kneeling on one knee and, keeping her low back straight, has lifted him onto her left knee.

student from a floor mat into a wheelchair. No one should attempt to lift a heavy impaired person alone. If there is doubt whether a student can be handled by one person, a second should be asked to help. Always plan a lift before proceeding.

Summarized on the following pages are methods that have been found helpful in lifting students. In describing these methods, we shall assume that the student is in a backlying position on a floor mat. Note, also, that this chapter concentrates only on lifting activity. Wheelchair transfers are covered in Chapter 13. Most lifting is done by classroom personnel in the school setting. Obviously, the techniques are equally applicable to nursing home attendants, parents, nursing staff, other support staff, and anyone else who may encounter a situation where lifting an impaired person is required. For the sake of brevity, the term "aide" is used in the remainder of this chapter to denote the person(s) doing the lifting.

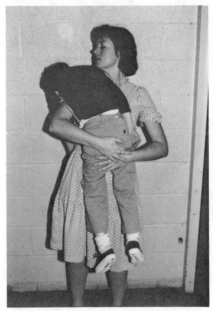

Figure 12.6. Correct carrying. A teacher carries one of her students close to her body to avoid back strain.

One-Person Lift

For a one-person lift, the instructional aide or teacher kneels on one knee facing the impaired student on the mat. One arm is wrapped behind the student's shoulders to cradle the neck in the bend of the aide's elbow. The aide's other arm is placed under the student's knees (see Figure 12.5). The student is lifted to rest on the aide's free knee; then the aide rises slowly to a standing position, keeping the student close to the body. Remember—the low back should be kept as vertical as possible while lifting. If the student experiences extensor thrust (see Chapter 10), the aide should proceed as indicated above, except bend the impaired student's neck forward and roll the shoulders slightly toward the aide before beginning to lift.

Two-Person Lifts

Two-person lifts may be accomplished by either the side-by-side or back-and-leg methods. We recommend using the side-by-side

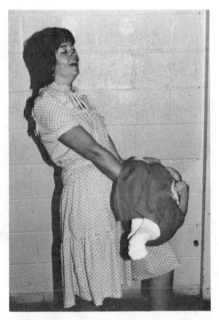

Figure 12.7. Incorrect carrying. The strain in trying to hold a student away from the body while carrying is evident in this photograph.

method whenever possible since the impaired student's weight is distributed equally between those making the lift. However, if space is limited or if there will be a need to make tight turns, the back-and-leg method permits more maneuverability.

Side-by-side Method Aides face each other, kneeling on one knee, on each side of the impaired person. Each places one arm diagonally behind the student's shoulders from the point of the near shoulder to below the far armpit (aides' arms cross on the student's back) (Figure 12.8). Aides' other arms go under the student's knees as in a one-person lift. The student is lifted; the aides shift their weight (free knee forward); and the student is rested on the aides' knees. Then, they rise to a standing position, keeping close together so that the student remains tight to their bodies. This method allows an equal portion of the student's weight to be borne by each person performing the lift.

Back-and-leg Method Kneeling at the student's head, the first aide places both arms under the student's arms so that the aide's

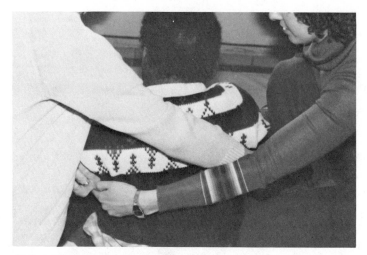

Figure 12.8. Side-by-side lifting method. The aides have crossed arms diagonally behind the student's shoulders in order to accomplish the lift.

hands are on the front of the student's chest. A second aide kneels on one knee parallel to the student's legs and locks both hands under the student's knees (Figure 12.9). Both then rise (using a count of one-two-three will help ensure that both lift together) and carry the

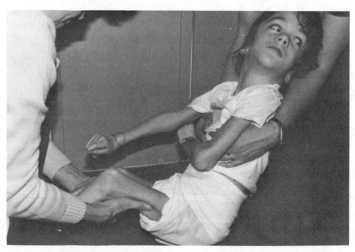

Figure 12.9. Back-and-leg lifting method. One aide lifts this student's chest while the other supports both knees. The aides work in unison to accomplish this lift.

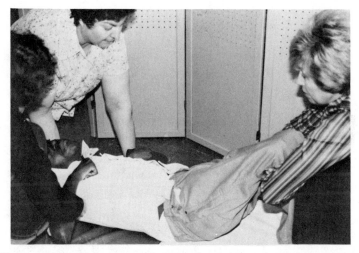

Figure 12.10. Three-person lift. Instructional aides assist the teacher in performing a three-person lift on one of their heavy students.

student in this manner. This method is particularly useful when an impaired student must be moved around an object such as a table or wheelchair. Aides should take turns lifting students' torsos so that the task of bearing the heavier load is shared equally.

Three-Person Lift

Two aides face each other, kneeling on one knee, on each side of the student, with a third at the student's feet. The first two aides cross arms in back of the student as in the side-by-side method. Their free hands may be used to support the student's waist or low back. The third aide supports the legs, usually by locking arms around the student's thighs (Figure 12.10). The lift is accomplished by the three working in unison to a one-two-three count. This lift is recommended for extremely heavy persons and for those who have severe scoliosis deformities.

Hydraulic Lifts

If hydraulic lifts are available, they should be used to move severely impaired persons. Hydraulic lifts are frequently found on special education buses and sometimes on vans and similar vehicles. Hand-operated hydraulic lifts (Figure 12.11) also are available at moderate

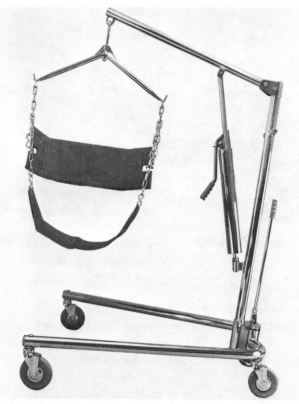

Figure 12.11. Hydraulic lift. If available, hydraulic lifts should be used to move heavy impaired persons. The lift pictured is available from Invacare Corporation. (Photograph courtesy of Invacare Corporation.)

cost. They are suitable for use in classrooms, nursing homes, and private residences. However, they are bulky and generally are not included as standard classroom equipment. Hand-operated hydraulic lifts are not portable and do not usually accompany an impaired individual during travel. As a result, there will be situations where the manual lifting methods emphasized in this chapter will be needed.

CONCLUSION

These lifting methods described in this chapter have proved to be instrumental in keeping student and staff injuries to a minimum.

Readers should be certain they understand the basic principles of body mechanics and how to execute these lifts properly before attempting to move a severely impaired person. Remember, too, to always use two or three people to perform a lift when one person may not be enough to ensure the safety of both the impaired person and the lifter.

REFERENCES

Finnie, N.R. *Handling the young cerebral palsied child at home*. New York: E.P. Dutton & Co., 1975.

Millen, H.M. *Body mechanics and safe transfer techniques*. Detroit: Aronsson Printing, 1974.

Wheelchairs and Transportation for Severely Impaired Persons

13

Wheelchairs for severely impaired persons serve an extensive role beyond merely providing mobility. Some are specially designed to correct or maintain body posture. Others have features to control abnormal reflex activity, and positioning devices to help prevent deformity. Adding a tray allows use of the chair for feeding and educational activities. The wheelchair provides a foundation upon which a management program can be built to meet school, home, and transportation needs.

It is the attending physician's responsibility to decide on the most appropriate type of wheelchair for an impaired person. Frequently, however, a doctor will seek the advice of physical and occupational therapists before making this decision. Also, parents and care providers often are called upon to provide background information about the impaired person's activities and environment. The doctor or therapist may consider the following kinds of questions:

What type of motor vehicle will be used to transport the person—compact car, large car, cab, van, school bus?

Will it be necessary to fold the chair for storage or travel?

Is there adequate room in the home for a large wheelchair?

Will the wheelchair need to accommodate a communication device?

When selecting a wheelchair for a student, a group approach to the decision, which allows for parental, nursing home, therapeutic, medical, and teaching input, is advisable. Indeed, many hospitals and schools are establishing wheelchair clinics where the responsibility for wheelchair selection is shared by those concerned with the impaired person (Riani & McNeny, 1981). Group members evaluate the impaired person's postural and mobility needs, identify the type of wheelchair most appropriate for the person, select a specific manufacturer, observe the person in a trial wheelchair, and take measurements of both the person and the wheelchair. Finally, the physician prescribes the appropriate chair. When possible, prescribing a commercially available chair as opposed to a custom-made chair is often preferable to help contain costs. At schools with a large population of wheelchair-bound students, wheelchairs in different styles and sizes can be borrowed for trial fittings. Once a prescribed wheelchair is purchased, it should be adjusted by the attending therapists to suit the user's impairments. It is extremely important to purchase the wheelchair from a vendor who will service the chair.

It is important that parents and primary care providers understand the working mechanism, care, and maintenance of the impaired person's wheelchair. The therapists involved in the selection process or the wheelchair salesperson can provide necessary information. These matters are most appropriately handled on an individual basis. However, an overview of the subject can provide useful background knowledge.

TYPES OF WHEELCHAIRS

Anyone who comes into contact with severely impaired persons—even on a casual basis—should be familiar with the kinds of wheelchairs used and should have practical knowledge of patient handling

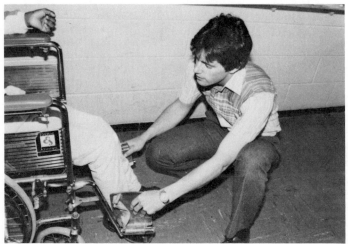

Figure 13.1. Foot plates. A teacher of the visually impaired makes sure that foot plates are folded in a vertical position before assisting his student out of the wheelchair.

and wheelchair operation and maintenance. Several kinds of chairs are discussed in the following paragraphs, including standard, travel, stroller, car seat, combination bed/chair, and power wheelchair. (Customized seating systems are discussed in Chapter 7.)

Standard Wheelchairs

Most readers will be familiar with the standard type wheelchair (see Figure 13.2). These chairs have wheel locking mechanisms located at the sides of the chair. When the lever is pushed toward the front of the chair, the lock is engaged. The chair should always be locked and the foot rest folded in the vertical position before placing an impaired person in or removing the individual from the chair (Figure 13.1). Some chairs are equipped with swinging, detachable leg rests. If present, the leg rests should be released and swung toward the back of the chair (Figure 13.2). Others may have elevating leg rests. These should be lowered to a position perpendicular to the floor, and the attached footrests folded up in order to allow room for the impaired person and attendant to stand in front of the chair.

Impaired persons who use a standard type wheelchair often are capable of supporting some weight on their feet. Those who can do so

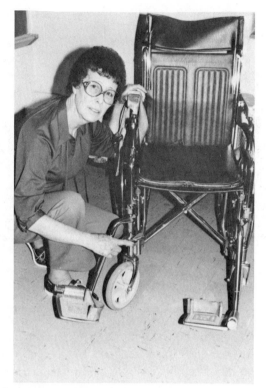

Figure 13.2. Swinging detachable leg rests. This instructional aide points to the lever that releases the leg rests.

should be encouraged to assist in transferring into the chair. First, position the person in front of the chair with the back of his or her legs touching the edge of the chair seat. Then, place an arm around the impaired person's back and guide him or her into a sitting position.

Travel Wheelchairs

Travel wheelchairs originally were developed to serve young handi-capped children as both therapeutic wheelchair and car seat. The rear wheels retract, and the back of the chair may be placed against a car's seat (Figures 13.3, 13.4, 13.5). As this type of chair gained popu-larity, larger models were manufactured to accommodate adolescents and adults. The larger chairs recline, but are not designed to be used as car seats. The back of the wheelchair is lowered by releasing the

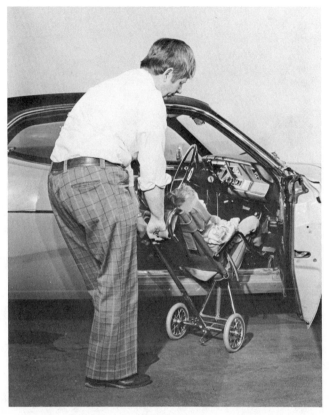

Figure 13.3.   Travel wheelchair. A child's father reclines the chair and places the front wheels into the car. (Photograph courtesy of Ortho-Kinetics, Inc.)

locking mechanism located just under the handlebars. The larger travel chairs offer more postural support and stability than most standard wheelchairs and are used by severely physically impaired persons whose needs fall between the standard and bed wheelchairs. Large travel chairs frequently are used in conjunction with van travel.

Strollers

Lightweight folding strollers (Figure 13.6) are designed to provide temporary transportation for handicapped children. Such strollers play an important part in the life of many impaired children. Their ease of use allows these children to be included in more social

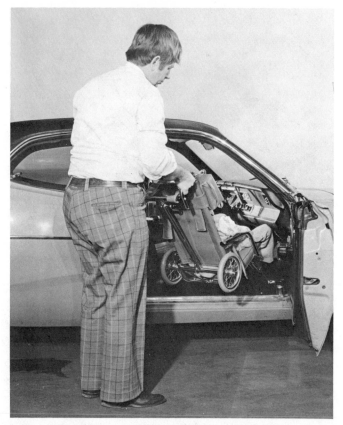

Figure 13.4. Travel wheelchair. The father retracts the rear wheels and lifts the chair into the car's front seat. (Photograph courtesy of Ortho-Kinetics, Inc.)

activities and outings. Although the basic stroller offers little, if any, postural correction, a foot rest, head rest, and firm back and seat insert may be added to provide support for moderately or severely impaired individuals. Strollers are especially useful for ambulatory children whose walking endurance is limited because of cardiac problems.

Car Seats

Car seats (Figure 13.7) may be placed either in the front or back seat of a car. The child is then put in the car seat with harness straps placed around each shoulder, between the legs, and over the lap. It is

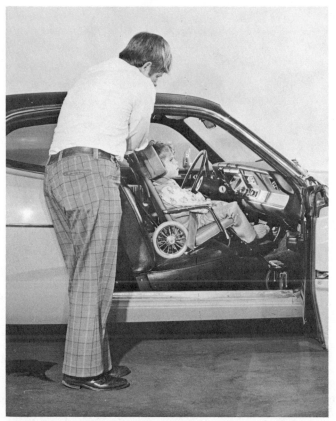

Figure 13.5. Travel wheelchair. The handlebars of the chair rest against the back of the car seat and the car safety belt is placed around the child and the travel chair. Travel wheelchairs are available from Ortho-Kinetics, Inc. (Photograph courtesy of Ortho-Kinetics, Inc.)

necessary to buckle the standard car safety belt around the car seat and child to hold them securely during travel. Car seats used with severely impaired persons are basically the same as the better quality safety seats used with normal children.

Bed Wheelchairs

Bed wheelchairs (Figure 13.8) are designed mainly for severely deformed adolescent and adult institutionalized persons. The chair consists of a multipositional bed attached to a standard wheelchair

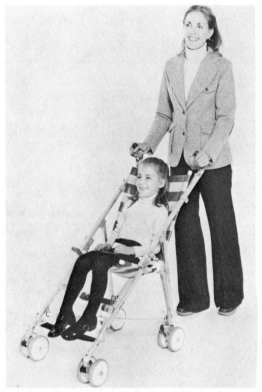

Figure 13.6. Folding stroller. The Pogon Transporter is a popular stroller. It provides temporary transportation for some severely impaired persons and for other less handicapped children. It is available from Genac Incorporated. (Photo courtesy of Genac Incorporated.)

frame. The wheel locking mechanism is similar to that of a standard wheelchair and is activated by a lever located near the wheels. The back of the chair is positioned by a bar that fits into slotted brackets. To adjust the chair back, it is usually best to have two aides on hand. Also, because the bed wheelchair is large and bulky, it is helpful to have one aide push the handlebars while a second guides the front of the chair when moving it in tight quarters.

Power Wheelchairs

Many severely impaired persons have begun to use power wheelchairs. Recent advances in postural support adaptations and oper-

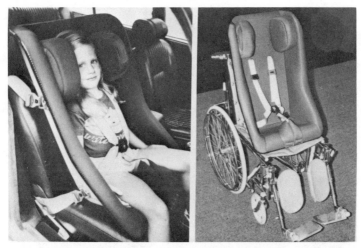

Figure 13.7. Car seat. This car seat is designed for transporting a child with limited head and trunk control in a car or bus. It is available from Childsafe Company and passes all U.S. Federal safety standards for crash testing of child restraints. A custom folding stroller base is also available from Childsafe Company so that the car seat can double as a wheelchair. (Photograph courtesy of Childsafe Company.)

ational control mechanisms make it possible for them to use such a chair safely (Trefler, Hand, Higgins, Chiarizzo, & Hobson, 1979). Although readers probably have observed persons using power wheelchairs in public, they may not be familiar with the details of operation and maintenance. Parents and staff should sit in the power wheelchair to be used by the student and learn to operate the controls. By knowing how to operate the chair, they will appreciate the skill and judgment needed for a student to use a chair safely, and be better able to help the student as he or she is learning to use the chair. Safe driving skills are important for the safety of the person in the chair and for others.

Power Wheelchair Driver's Test Students should pass a power wheelchair driver's test before they are allowed to operate a power wheelchair independently at school. One such test that was developed by the authors in conjunction with occupational therapist Mary Jo Kurily is described in the following paragraphs. This test consists of six skill levels that have been designed to evaluate the student's ability to operate a power wheelchair successfully.

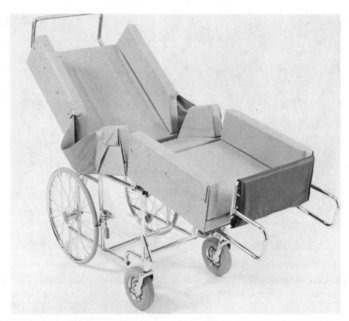

Figure 13.8. Bed wheelchair. This multipositional bed wheelchair allows severely impaired persons to be positioned in either a reclined or upright position. It is available from Everest & Jennings. (Photograph courtesy of Everest & Jennings.)

1. ***Basic operation*** Basic operation includes turning the control switch on and off, and moving the chair forward, forward right, forward left, backward, backward right, and backward left for a short distance (less than 3 feet).
2. ***Half turns*** Half turns involve maneuvering the chair 90 degrees right or left and then continuing forward for a short distance (less than 3 feet).
3. ***Full turns*** Full turns (180 degrees) require reversal of direction by pivoting the chair right or left and then continuing forward in one sustained motion.
4. ***Obstacle course*** The obstacle course requires that the student maneuver the wheelchair in a hallway or classroom, avoiding both stationary obstructions (trash baskets, chairs) and moving objects (people, other wheelchairs).
5. ***Doorways*** The student must maneuver through a series of doorways, approaching from straight ahead, right, and left. The

student first learns to drive the chair through wide or double doorways, then advances to narrow or single doorways.

6. *Ramps* The student must climb and descend short ramps. This is the most difficult wheelchair training task since it requires that the student judge distance on an inclined or declined narrow surface.

Each skill level must be mastered fully before the student is permitted to progress to a more difficult task. Students must pass skill level 4 for independent classroom driving, skill level 5 for driving within the school building, and skill level 6 for driving in and out of school.

Power Wheelchair Operation Power chairs are recommended mainly for indoor use and are not designed for steep grades. They have a driving range of up to 25 miles depending upon the model of chair, size of patient, and speed (Everest & Jennings, 1977). They are operated either by hand control boxes (mounted on the right or the left armrest) or by chin or mouth controls. A joystick controls direction and, in some cases, speed. Usually, for a severely impaired patient, a control system involving a preset speed is used because it is the least complicated to operate. Some power wheelchairs have removable batteries so that the chair may be folded for transportation (A-BEC, 1976).

Power Wheelchair Maintenance It is important that care providers understand the maintenance procedures necessary to keep a power chair in good working order. The battery should be kept fully charged, which usually involves connecting the battery to an electric battery charger and plugging the charger into a wall outlet each night. Most battery chargers have an automatic cutoff when fully charged, making it safe to leave them plugged in overnight. However, *check* before doing so to avoid danger of explosion or fire. Battery water level should be checked every 2 weeks, and distilled water (regular tap water can damage the battery) should be added as needed to maintain the proper level. Be careful not to spill the liquid when opening battery cells. It is highly acidic and can burn skin and clothes. (Some newer batteries are sealed units that do not require periodic checking. The top of the battery indicates clearly whether this is the case.) Most power wheelchairs have pneumatic (inflatable) tires. These should be checked at least once a month and maintained

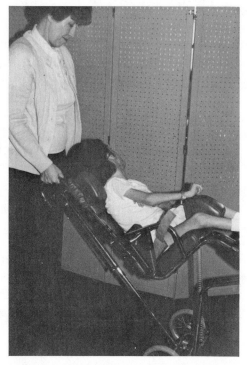

Figure 13.9. One-person positioning in wheelchair. This instructional aide tilts the travel chair backward, allowing gravity to pull the student back in the seat.

at the recommended pressure to ensure optimum wheelchair maneuverability. Tires should also be checked for signs of uneven wear. Poor alignment can cause steering problems.

A power wheelchair is an expensive and sophisticated piece of equipment. Proper care will prevent unnecessary repair cost.

POSITIONING IN WHEELCHAIRS

Positioning in a wheelchair is critical for a person's comfort and posture. Regardless of the type of wheelchair being used, it is important that the impaired person's buttocks be as far back in the chair as possible. One way to accomplish this is to tilt the chair backward and allow gravity to pull the impaired person into the seat (Figure 13.9). If two people are available to help with positioning,

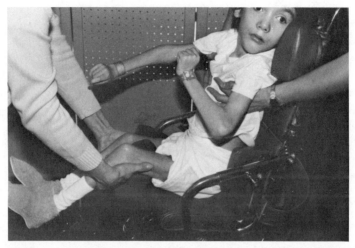

Figure 13.10. Two-person positioning in wheelchair. The student is lifted well back into his travel wheelchair.

one should stand behind the chair and, once the person is seated, wrap his or her arms under the impaired person's arms and around the front of the chest. The second should stand at the front of the wheelchair and grasp under the impaired person's knees. At the count of three, the two should lift the person well back into the chair (Figure 13.10).

Special wheelchair postural attachments such as scoliosis pads, abductor or adductor pads, and headrests (see Chapter 7) should only be adjusted by the attending therapist. Parents and care providers should keep the therapist informed of any problems with these attachments. Care providers should also check the nuts and bolts securing the attachment and tighten them periodically. Weekly checks of this type will help prevent the attachments from becoming lost or misaligned.

GENERAL CARE INSTRUCTIONS
FOR ALL KINDS OF WHEELCHAIRS

Many rules of wheelchair maintenance will seem obvious, but they can easily be overlooked if a conscientious attitude toward general care is not observed. The following general care instructions should be followed.

Never put a wheelchair in the shower or let it stand outside in the rain! Water will cause the wheels and metal parts of the chair frame to rust. Excessive exposure to moisture will ruin a wheelchair very quickly. If excess exposure to water cannot be avoided, a stainless steel wheelchair frame will be needed. Such frames add about 20% to the cost of a wheelchair, but are a money saver for long-term use in a moist environment since stainless steel will not rust. It is permissible (even helpful), however, to wash upholstered portions with a mild soap and water. Wheelchairs should be vacuumed daily to remove food crumbs from seams. Wheels should be oiled at least monthly. Commercial wheelchair cleaning is available at some dealer centers. A yearly deep cleaning of this type will help to keep the wheelchair in good condition and prolong its life. Remember, for severely impaired persons, wheelchairs become almost part of their person and should be kept clean and in good condition.

TIPS FOR TRANSPORTATION SAFETY

Because many severely impaired individuals have limited sitting balance, the following precautions should be observed to ensure safe travel in a wheelchair:

> Be sure that the person is sitting well back in the chair, and secure all safety belts before travel.
> Engage wheel brakes before lifting a wheelchair using a hydraulic platform.
> Two adults should accompany an impaired individual when he or she must negotiate a ramp or step—one in front of the chair and one behind it.
> Check the person frequently during travel to be sure that all restraints are clear of the neck area.
> Chairs should be locked securely into place if they are to be used to carry patients in moving vehicles.

REFERENCES

A-BEC, Inc. *Folding electric wheelchairs: A new dimension in mobility*. Torrence, CA: A-BEC, 1976.

Everest & Jennings, Inc. *Owners manual, indoor power driving model 3N*. Los Angeles: Everest & Jennings, 1977.

Riani, R.M., & McNeny, R. Wheelchair clinic: A better way to prescribe. *Clinical Management in Physical Therapy*, 1981, *1*(2), 18–19.

Trefler, D., Hand, S., Higgins, E., Chiarizzo, S., & Hobson, D. A modular seating system for cerebral-palsied children. *Developmental Medicine and Child Neurology*, 1979, *20*, 199–204.

Section IV

———

LOOKING AHEAD

New
Directions

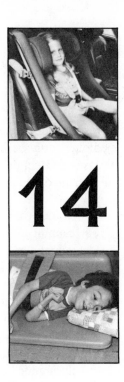

14

As indicated in the preceding chapters, managing persons with serious physical handicaps is a new frontier for health professionals, rehabilitation engineers, care providers, and educators. As such, there is ample opportunity for all concerned to contribute toward the evolution of better prevention and management programs that will help in the integration of persons with serious handicaps into society. The advances of today are exciting, the promises of tomorrow encouraging.

This chapter explores some of the possibilities for future progress in caring for seriously physically handicapped persons. Advances in technology and medicine, as well as changes in social consciousness, offer a brighter future for persons with physical handicaps. It is uplifting to speculate about that future.

SIZE OF THE SERIOUSLY
PHYSICALLY HANDICAPPED POPULATION

The size of the seriously physically handicapped population will obviously be of concern to those working to improve prevention and management programs. Many factors need to be considered before predicting whether the numbers of seriously handicapped people will increase or decrease in the next decade. Current developments in medicine could be interpreted to indicate a drastic decrease in such diseases and conditions (Sternfeld & Berenberg, 1982). These developments include the following:

> Methods (for instance, amniocentesis) for detecting handicapping of the fetus during early pregnancy are being developed and refined. With accurate information and genetic counseling, some parents will undoubtedly limit the size of their families or consider the option of legal therapeutic abortion, made available by the U.S. Supreme Court.
>
> Use of ultrasound is becoming widespread in identifying dangerous situations of late pregnancy. In such cases, doctors may perform a Caesarean section to avoid damage to the baby during the birth process, or may induce the delivery sooner if fetal distress is detected.
>
> Treatment of the fetus is becoming increasingly possible during pregnancy. For example, doctors now are able to drain excess cerebrospinal fluid before the infant is born, thus preventing hydrocephalus. Administration of medicine to the fetus is also possible in certain instances.
>
> Improvements in intensive care for newborn babies of low birth weight are bringing about greater success in preventing brain damage in these infants.
>
> Vaccines are likely to be developed in the near future that will be effective in preventing meningitis, and, in turn, the incidence of brain damage and related physical handicaps caused by the associated complications of meningitis (Sternfeld & Berenberg, 1982).
>
> New drugs are being developed to treat viral infections of the central nervous system.

Countering these positive developments, however, are other current trends that will serve to swell the number of seriously handicapped persons:

All of us are increasingly exposed to hazardous environmental substances that can produce long-term genetic damage and cause direct fetal brain damage.

The prevalence of drug, alcohol, and other substance abuse raises the risk of fetal damage.

Trends toward both earlier- and later-life births increase the risks for both mother and baby.

Reduced availability of prenatal care, in part a reflection of budget-related cuts in social programs, will mean that some mothers are less prepared to deliver healthy infants.

Right-to-life legislation may considerably limit the availability of therapeutic abortions.

Child abuse continues to grow and is a problem for which society has not found a solution.

The number and severity of personal injury automobile accidents, after declining somewhat in the late 1970s, is expected to increase dramatically as cars get smaller and provide less crash protection.

The life span of severely impaired persons will continue to increase.

Unfortunately, the positive medical advances may not offset fully the factors tending to increase the future numbers of severely impaired persons. This means that the number of seriously handicapped persons is likely to remain at least at its present level and may even increase somewhat over the next decade.

SOCIAL ATTITUDES AND COST CONTAINMENT

Society will most likely continue—even strengthen—its efforts toward deinstitutionalization, normalization, and education of physically impaired persons, coupled with a greater awareness and understanding of these persons by the general public. However, the pursuit of cost-effectiveness may well have a major impact on determining how these goals are achieved. A shorter period of formal education could perhaps be one option considered for severely impaired persons, in conjunction with a less expensive maintenance-type program for those who are not capable of participating in sheltered workshops. At the time this book was written, an attempt to limit the principles of PL 94-142 had met with such widespread opposition from a concerned public and Congress that the proposed changes were withdrawn. It may be some time before this issue is raised again.

Regardless, cost-effectiveness will inevitably become more of a consideration in providing therapy to handicapped persons. Present and prospective research is likely to result in improved and more realistic therapeutic management of severely impaired persons. Compatible with this development should be continued refinement and general acceptance of the team approach to physical therapy/orthopaedic care of seriously physically handicapped persons.

TECHNOLOGY

The technological advances from which persons with physical handicaps will benefit will be numerous. New, lightweight materials are coming to the attention of rehabilitation engineers. These will be fashioned into a variety of customized seating systems and positioning aides for severely impaired persons that will be available at a relatively low cost. Significant benefits in terms of both individual comfort and mobility may be expected.

It also appears likely that electrical devices will be attached to the body to help balance muscles in neuromuscularly and severely impaired persons. For example, electrical stimulation, presently used in the control of idiopathic scoliosis (Chapter 7), may have future application for those with spastic neuromuscular conditions. Such devices may replace corsets and braces as the preferred means for preventing or delaying deformity.

Advances in electronics and microcomputers will enable even the most severely physically impaired person to use a communication system. As these systems are technologically refined, the cost of such systems, it is hoped, will be lowered to the point where they can be used by most handicapped persons. Perhaps with less need for bracing mechanisms, insurance providers will accept communication systems as necessary equipment for nonverbal persons and expand their coverage to cover purchase costs.

ADVANCES IN MEDICAL CARE

Electronic and radiological advances will aid the physician greatly in diagnosing and prognosticating the disease process. The computerized tomography (CT) scanner is just the beginning of a host of electronic and radiological imaging. Particularly for problems related to the central nervous system, physicians increasingly will use CT scanners to unlock secrets of the brain and its blood supply during a variety of different states. At present, variations of positron emission tomography (PET) scanners are used experimentally to examine chemical processing within the brain itself. The information obtained from these studies undoubtly will lead to much improved diagnostic acumen.

Computerized electronic gait laboratories are providing physicians and physical therapists with a better understanding of muscle function in spastic patients. This information is especially helpful to orthopaedic surgeons in preoperative assessment, in surgical planning, and in determining the success of surgical procedures. Physical therapists also use the electronic information provided by the gait laboratory to plan and monitor gait training and pre- and postoperative exercise programs. At present, gait laboratories are used with moderately and mildly handicapped persons with great success. In the future, highly technical gait analyses should produce spin-off information about oxygen utilization and exercise that doctors and therapists can apply to the severely impaired population.

In summary, electronic and radiological technology will enable both doctors and physical therapists to make better use of their resources in managing the neuromuscular problems of seriously handicapped persons.

ADVANCES IN SURGICAL CARE

Many of the surgical techniques used today were described and performed by doctors at the turn of the century. Since that time, however, numerous improvements in those techniques have evolved, allowing for greater refinement of surgical practices and successful new operations. Further advances in present technical aspects of surgery to prevent, correct, or limit physical impairments are not likely. However, patient selection, timing, appropriateness, and benefits from surgery will be improved by a more detailed and sophisticated look at the patients pre- and postoperatively. Much of this information will be obtained by use of electronic computer analysis.

In addition, surgical techniques will be adapted for severely impaired persons. For example, the Luque instrumentation for surgical control of scoliosis mentioned in Chapter 7 should prove extremely helpful to severely impaired persons since this surgical procedure requires no brace or cast postoperatively. Also, earlier use of surgery, prior to formation of severe spinal curvatures, will provide neuromuscularly and severely involved persons better and long-term correction of potentially serious spinal deformities.

In the future, reduced periods of postoperative immobilization and improved postoperative management can be expected to reduce surgical risks for neuromuscularly and severely impaired persons. Certainly, doctors will achieve a better understanding of the disease process and its natural history through modern technology. This will enable surgeons to take a more aggressive approach to prevention of deformity via surgery and achievement of more successful surgical results.

CONCLUSION

The most significant changes to occur over the next 10 years will likely involve replacing or refining current technology used to control muscle imbalances. As these changes occur, it is hoped that many of the techniques for dealing with physical handicaps discussed in this book will become outdated. Better, more technologically advanced and successful techniques will replace them. Even so, the need for a team management philosophy—the philosophy of management that has been interwoven throughout this book—will endure. Such a management approach to the care of seriously handicapped persons will contribute toward making their lives and the lives of those who take care of them easier, happier, and more productive.

REFERENCES

Sternfeld, L., & Berenberg, W. Twenty-five years of cerebral palsy research. *American Academy for Cerebral Palsy and Developmental Medicine News*, 1982, *102*, 33, 2–3.

APPENDICES

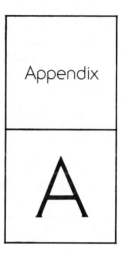

Appendix

A

Glossary

Abduction   Sideways movement of the limbs (arms and/or legs) away from the middle of the body.

Acetabulum   A cup-shaped cavity in the hip. The acetabulum (meaning little cup) serves as a ''socket'' for the ''ball''-shaped head of the thigh bone (femur).

Achilles tendon   The fibrous cord connecting the muscle located at the back of the calf to a bone in the back of the foot. The Achilles tendon was named for the Greek hero whose mother held him by the ankle to dip him in the river Styx to make him invincible, leaving him vulnerable only in this area. It is also referred to as the heel cord.

Acquired   Refers to conditions produced by influences originating outside the person—not genetic in origin.

Adduction   Sideways movement of the limbs (arms and/or legs) toward the midline of the body.

Ambulation   The act of walking or moving about.

Anterior   Toward the front of the body.

Arthritis   A general term used to describe a variety of conditions in which pain and inflammation occur in and around joints.

Arthrodesis The surgical fixation of a joint.

Asphyxia A condition caused by lack of air in the lungs—suffocation.

Asymmetrical tonic neck reflex (ATNR) An automatic reflexive action in which turning the head sideways causes straightening of the arm and leg on the side of the body toward which the face is turned and bending of the arm and leg on the opposite side of the body.

Ataxia Irregularity of muscle action; incoordination of voluntary muscular movement; e.g., wide base, staggering gait.

Athetosis Repeated slow, purposeless involuntary motions, especially severe in the hands.

Atrophy A wasting away; a reduction in the size of a cell, tissue, muscle, organ, or body part.

Augmentative communication systems Aids, such as communication boards or gestures, that enhance or add to a nonspeaking person's ability to communicate.

Behavior modification Techniques designed to alter existing behavior in some predetermined manner.

Biceps Muscle located on the front of the upper arm.

Body mechanics The use of correct and efficient movements of the human body to perform a purposeful act.

Bony surgery The surgical cutting of bone to realign or fuse a joint.

Calcaneus Heel bone.

Calcaneus deformity A condition in which the forefoot is pulled upward and the heel downward.

Central nervous system The part of the nervous system primarily responsible for controlling voluntary motion and thought processes. It is comprised of the brain and spinal cord.

Cerebral palsy A condition involving disabilities in movement and posture that result from damage to the brain before or during birth, or in infancy.

Cerebrospinal fluid A liquid that flows inside and outside the brain and in the spinal column. It protects the central nervous system from sudden pressure changes and provides nutrients. Normal cerebrospinal fluid is clear, colorless, and odorless.

Cervical A term pertaining to the neck.

Circumduction A smooth coordinated circular movement that revolves around a given joint; a movement that contains elements of flexion, abduction, extension, and adduction.

Cognitive   Refers to the act or process of perceiving or knowing.

Concave   Refers to an inwardly rounded curve; e.g. the interior shape of a ball.

Congenital   Refers to conditions that are present at birth, regardless of their causation. These conditions may originate before or at birth.

Contracture   A permanent shortening of a muscle-tendon unit (muscle, tendon, and/or joint capsule) due to spasticity or paralysis, resulting in less than normal range of motion of a joint.

Convexity   An outwardly rounded curve; e.g., the exterior shape of a ball.

Cranial sutures   A type of fibrous joint found in the skull in which opposed joint surfaces are separated at birth, allowing the skull to expand and the brain to grow. The opposing surfaces gradually grow together, becoming closely knit and thereafter immovable.

Decubitus ulcer   An ulcer of the skin commonly called a bedsore.

Degenerative disease   A condition or illness characterized by progression from a higher to a lower level of body function.

Deinstitutionalization   The name given a movement to eliminate large impersonal facilities where mentally retarded and handicapped persons reside. Alternatives to institutionalization involve a handicapped or retarded person remaining within the family unit or residing in a small group home.

Developmental age   The age in months at which an individual can perform a specific action. For example, a child normally learns to stand independently at about 12 months of age. If a 15-year-old person just learned this skill, he or she would be considered to be functioning at a 12-month developmental age level in relation to this skill.

Diathermy   A therapeutic treatment in which the body tissues are heated by means of an oscillating electromagnetic field of high frequency; a dry heat.

Diplegia   Muscle involvement of similar parts of the body, e.g., legs.

Dislocation   A term applied to a joint to indicate that the surfaces of the bones that form it are no longer in contact or are displaced.

Distal   Away from the center of the body or a point of reference.

Dorsiflex   A backward bending of the hand at the wrist, or lifting of the forefoot.

Down's syndrome   A condition characterized by a flat face, small, low-bridged nose, upward slanted folds of skin at the inner corners of the eyes, and moderate mental deficiency associated with chromosomal abnormality. Down's syndrome is diagnosed by chromosomal studies and identified as trisomy 21.

Duchenne muscular dystrophy A hereditary and progressive body weakness found only in boys that is caused by degeneration of muscle fibers.

Dysplasia Abnormal development of a body part.

Encephalopathy Any degenerative disease of the brain.

Equinus A likeness to a horse's leg.

Equinus deformity A condition in which the heel of the foot is pulled upward and the forefoot downward.

Esophageal reflux A backward or return flow of food up the tube (esophagus) extending from the mouth to the stomach.

Etiology The cause or origins of a disease or abnormal condition; also theory and study of the factors that cause diseases or abnormal conditions.

Eversion Movement of the foot in which the sole turns outward away from the midline of the body.

Expressive language The ability to speak, to produce symbolic gestures, and/or to write.

Extension The straightening of a joint, which diminishes the angle between bones that meet in the joint; the opposite of flexion.

Extensor thrust A reaction in which the neck, back, hips, and knees extend or straighten causing the body to arch backward.

Femur The thigh bone, extending from the pelvis to the knee.

Fine motor skills Activities using the smaller muscles in the body, such as functional hand activities.

Flexion The bending of a joint; the opposite of extension.

Floppy infant A descriptive term used to refer to children (age 1 month to 12–14 months) affected by a nonspecific, congenital muscle, nerve, or brain disease characterized by muscle weakness and low muscle tone.

Fracture The breaking of a part, usually a bone.

Functional spinal curve A supple abnormal curve or exaggeration of a normal curve of the spine that may be corrected by application of some type of force, such as a brace, traction, or physical manipulation or simple positioning.

Gait The manner of style of walking.

Gestural language The use of hand motions to form a sign representing a word; a sign method of communication.

Goniometer An instrument for measuring angles.

Gross motor Activities using the larger muscles in the body; e.g., head control, creeping, sitting, standing, running.

Head lag A lack of head control in which the head falls backward into extension when the subject is pulled from a backlying position into a sitting position. This is normal in newborns, but is abnormal after 2–3 months of life.

Heel cord The tendon of the muscle located at the back of the calf from the knee to the heel.

Hemiplegia Paralysis of one side of the body; muscular abnormality of an arm and leg on one side of the body.

Hiatal hernia A protrusion of any structure through the esophageal opening of the diaphragm.

Hip adductors A group of muscles located on the inside of the thigh; primarily responsible for a sideways movement of the leg toward the midline.

Humerus The bone that extends from the shoulder to the elbow.

Hydrocephalus A neurological condition in which an abnormal amount of spinal fluid accumulates in and around the brain. The excess fluid can cause increased pressure on the brain and, in the young, enlargement in the circumference of the skull.

Hydrotherapy The application of water in the treatment of disease.

Hypermobility Excessive elasticity of joints that allows them to move beyond their normal limits.

Hypertonia A condition involving excessive response to stimuli (tone) by skeletal muscles.

Hypotonia A condition of diminished tone of skeletal muscles.

Idiopathic Of unknown causation.

Incontinence Inability to control bowel and bladder activity.

Inferior Pertaining to a lower segment, usually of the body or a body part.

Inversion Movement of the foot in which the sole turns toward the midline of the body.

Inward rotation Turning or rotating a limb toward the midline of the body.

Kyphosis An abnormally increased backward curvature of the spine that causes a hump-like appearance of the upper back in a pathological state. Kyphosis also describes the normal backward curve of the thoracic spine when viewed from the side.

Lamina   A general term for a thin flat plate or layer, usually referring to the posterior of the vertebrae.

Landouzy-Dejerine muscular dystrophy   A form of a hereditary and progressive body weakness caused by degeneration of muscle fibers that has its onset in adolescence and progresses slowly.

Lateral   Pertaining to or toward the sides of the body.

Lordosis   An abnormally increased forward curvature of the spine that causes a "hollow" or "sway" appearance of the lower back in a pathological state. Lordosis also describes the normal forward curve of the "sway" appearance of the lower back.

Lower extremity   A term used to describe the thigh, leg, and foot.

Lumbar   Pertaining to the low back.

Macrocephalic   An abnormally large head size.

Mainstreaming   Placement of a handicapped student in a school situation in which he or she may participate in any or all of the regular education programs and activities.

Medial   Pertaining to or toward the midline of the body.

Meninges   Membranes that envelop the brain and spinal cord.

Meningitis   An inflammation of the membranes that envelop the brain and spinal cord.

Meningocele   A protrusion of the meninges through a defect in the skull or vertebral column.

Metabolic diseases   Abnormal conditions that involve chemical processes within the body.

Microcephaly   A condition involving an abnormally small head.

Midline   An imaginary line drawn from head to toes that separates the body into right and left halves.

Monoplegia   Paralysis of a limb.

Moro reflex   An automatic response that is triggered by sudden removal of support while a person is being lowered from a sitting position to a backlying position.

Motor abilities   Meaningful bodily activities, produced by the interaction of muscles, nerves, and joints, such as rolling, sitting, creeping, standing, and walking.

Movement dysfunction   Abnormal motion of any body part, a limb, limbs, or the entire body.

Multiple sclerosis   A progressive disease of the central nervous system characterized by patchy lesions along the protective sheath of certain nerves.

Muscle tone   The degree of vigor or tension in skeletal muscles.

Muscular dystrophy   A group of genetically caused, degenerative diseases of the muscles characterized by weakness and atrophy.

Musculoskeletal conditions   Conditions affecting the muscles or bones, or both.

Myelomeningocele   Protrusion of the spinal cord through a defect in the vertebral canal.

Natal   Pertaining to birth.

Neonatal   Pertaining to the first 4 weeks after birth.

Neurological conditions   Conditions pertaining to the nervous system.

Normalization   A principle stating that treatment and services for handicapped persons should be provided in such a manner as to enable them to reside as close as possible to a normal setting within a given society.

Obturator nerve   A cordlike structure comprised of a collection of nerve fibers that conveys impulses between the central nervous system and the hip adductor muscles.

Occupational therapist   A health professional skilled in the provision of creative activity designed to promote recovery or rehabilitation of the body's small muscles following accident or disease.

Opisthotonos   Severe muscle spasms causing a person to bend backward like a bow.

Orthopaedist   A medical doctor (surgeon) specializing in the treatment of bones, joints, and muscles.

Orthosis   An appliance or apparatus used to correct, prevent, support, or align deformities or to improve function of movable body parts.

Orthotist   A person especially trained in making prescribed orthoses and tailoring orthoses to meet an individual's needs.

Os calcis   Alternative name for the calcaneus or large bone of the hindfoot or heel.

Osteogenesis imperfecta   An inherited condition in which the bones are abnormally brittle and easily fractured.

Outward rotation   Turning or rotating of a limb away from the midline of the body.

Paraplegia   Paralysis of both legs and the lower portion of the trunk.

Patella   The knee cap, a small bone situated at the front of the knee.

Pathological   Pertaining to a disease.

Pedorthist   A trained specialist who constructs shoes or other apparatuses used to support, align, prevent, or correct foot deformities.

Pelvic obliquity   A slanting or inclination of the pelvis such that it is not positioned in a horizontal plane when the person is standing or sitting.

Perineal   The pelvic floor or diaper area.

Physical therapist   A licensed health professional who plans and administers physical treatment programs for medically referred patients to restore function, relieve pain, and prevent disability of the body's limbs and large muscles following disease, injury, or loss of body part.

Plantar grasp reflex   An automatic curling of the toes when pressure is applied to the ball of the foot.

Plantigrade position   The normal standing or walking attitude of the human foot, such that weight is distributed across the full sole of the foot.

Poliomyelitis   A disease caused by a virus that attacks nerve tissue in the spinal cord or cranial nerves, or both, and may result in muscular weakness or paralysis.

Posterior   Toward the back of the body.

Postnatal   After birth.

Postural reflex   An automatic response to a stimulus that results in a change of attitude of the body.

Prenatal   Before birth.

Prognosis   A forecast as to the probable outcome of a disease or condition.

Pronation   Movement in the forearm that results in turning the palm downward.

Prone   A person lying horizontally on the abdomen with the face turned downward (facelying).

Protective extension   A reaction to loss of sitting or standing balance in which the arms straighten to prevent injury to the head.

Proximal   Closer to any point of reference.

Quadriceps   A group of muscles located on the front of the upper leg which flex the hip and extend the knee.

Quadriplegia   Paralysis of all four limbs.

Radial deviation   Motion, occurring at the wrist, that causes a lateral movement of the hand toward the thumb side.

Range of motion   Exercise consisting of moving the parts of the body in specific ways.

Receptive language   The ability to understand spoken language.

Reflex   An involuntary response to a specific stimulus.

Remission   A lessening or disappearance of disease symptoms that usually is temporary in nature. Also, the period during which such an event occurs.

Rigidity   A stiffness or inflexibility of a body part.

Roentgenogram   Photography of various body parts by means of roentgen rays; an X ray.

Rotoscoliosis   A condition in which a sideways curve of the spine is coupled with a rotation of the ribs and vertebral bodies.

Rumination   Regurgitation of swallowed food followed by chewing another time.

Sandifer syndrome   A combination of **hiatal hernia** and abnormal posturing of the head and neck.

Scapula   A flat, triangular bone in the back of the shoulder—often called the shoulder blade.

Scissoring   Crossing of the legs with the knees straight.

Scoliosis   An abnormal sideways curvature of the spine.

Sepsis   The presence of bacterial infection in the blood or body tissues; blood poisoning.

Shunt   A surgically implanted tube that connects two blood vessels, two spaces, or two organs.

Sidelying   A position in which a person rests on either the right or left side of the body, usually with legs slightly bent.

Skeletal deformity   A distortion of the bones and joints.

Soft tissue surgery   Operations that involve lengthening muscles and tendons or releasing tight structures such as ligaments and capsules of joints.

Spasticity   Permanently increased muscle tone causing stiffness in movements.

Speech-language pathologist   A health professional specially trained and qualified to assist persons in overcoming speech and language disorders.

Spina bifida   A congenital defect of the body spinal column characterized by incomplete closure of the spinal bones during fetal development.

Spinous processes The projections on the back of the vertebrae.

Staggering reactions Movement (forward, backward, or sideways) of the feet that protects upright posture when the body's position in space is displaced by force.

Structural spinal curve A rigid abnormal spinal curvature involving permanent changes in alignment of the spinal vertebrae.

Subluxation A condition in which surfaces of the bones forming a joint begin to slip out of alignment.

Superior Pertains to an upper segment, usually of the body or a body part.

Supination Movement in the forearm that turns the palm upward.

Supine A person positioned horizontally on the back with the face upward (backlying).

Talus The bone of the foot that interacts with the tibia and fibula to form the ankle joint—often called the ankle bone.

Teratogenic agents Chemical or physical factors that produce physical defects in offspring during pregnancy.

Thoracic Pertaining to or affecting the body cavity that contains the heart and lungs.

Tibia The larger bone of the lower leg—the shin bone.

Trauma A wound or injury.

Tremor A rhythmic, involuntary movement of certain muscle groups.

Triceps The muscle located at the back of the upper arm. The triceps is primarily responsible for extending the elbow joint.

Triplegia Paralysis of three extremities.

Tube feeding Liquid nourishment administered by means of a tube inserted surgically through a constructed hole in a person's abdomen or inserted through the mouth or nose.

Ulnar deviation Movement at the wrist that causes a sideways motion of the hand away from the thumb.

Upper extremity Arm and forearm; shoulder through hand.

Valgus Bent outward; angulation of a part away from the midline.

Varus Bent inward; angulation of a part toward the midline.

Manufacturers/ Distributors of Prescriptive Equipment

<table>
<tr><td>Appendix</td></tr>
<tr><td>B</td></tr>
</table>

Selecting the most appropriate equipment for use by a seriously handicapped person is a challenging task for all concerned. It is virtually impossible for any individual to keep abreast of all commercially available products and their adaptations. Information may be obtained through national and community organizations, school and hospital resource libraries, equipment manufacturers, and the therapists and doctors working with the handicapped person.

In Michigan, handicapped persons and those concerned with their care may consult PAM (Physically Impaired Association of Michigan) Assistance Center for current equipment information. PAM Assistance Center's staff provides information about commercially available and adaptive equipment for personal care, clothing, recreation, and mobility for handicapped persons regardless of age or disability. Although this free service is directed to Michigan residents, inquiries from out-of-state persons are welcome. Interested readers may contact PAM Assistance Center, 601 W. Maple, Box 21037, Lansing, Michigan 48909, phone (517) 371-5897.

Prescriptive equipment and certain products that have been helpful in providing physical management programs for seriously handicapped persons have been mentioned throughout the text. For the reader's convenience, this appendix provides a list of the manufacturers/distributors of equipment discussed in the text and information about their product line.

Brookstone Company
127 Vose Farm Road
Peterborough, New Hampshire 03458
(603) 924-7181

> Brookstone carries hard-to-find tools that may be purchased by ordering through their catalog. Brookstone products are not designed for handicapped persons. However, some items, such as the headlight described in Chapter 11, may be used for special purposes with the severely impaired population.

Childsafe Company
P.O. Box 633
Pacific Palisades, California 90272
(213) 454-6612

> Childsafe Company carries bath and toileting aids, Rida chairs, car seats, and wheelchair inserts for handicapped children.

Danmar Products, Inc.
2390 Winewood
Ann Arbor, Michigan 48103
(313) 761-1990

> Danmar's special products include swim aids, protective head and face gear, and head, chest, and limb supports for impaired individuals.

Everest & Jennings Inc.
3233 E. Mission Oaks Blvd.
Camarillo, California 93010
(805) 987-6911

> In addition to a full line of wheelchairs, Everest & Jennings specializes in medical, rehabilitation, and health care products.

Fred Sammons, Inc.
Box 32
Brookfield, Illinois 60513–0032
1-800-323-7305

> Fred Sammons, Inc., offers a wide variety of self-help aids and orthotic supplies through catalog sales. These products are intended for professional use with and recommended for handicapped persons.

Freeman Manufacturing Co.
900 W. Chicago Road
Sturgis, Michigan 49091
(616) 651-2371

> Freeman Manufacturing Co. produces body supports, traction devices, and rehabilitation aids.

Genac Incorporated
1700 S. 120th Street
Lafayette, Colorado 80026
1-800-525-0364

> Genac Incorporated specializes in manufacturing lightweight stroller transportation for handicapped persons. Stroller sizes range from toddler to adult, and are available with posture support inserts.

Invacare Corporation
1200 Taylor Street
Elyria, Ohio 44035
(216) 365-9321

> Invacare Corporation produces a complete line of standard wheelchairs, walking aids, bath safety aids, and hydraulic lifts. Invacare products are distributed nationally through authorized dealers.

Medipedic, Inc.
P.O. Box 89
Jackson, Michigan 49204
(205) 647-0444

> Medipedic offers a complete selection of orthopaedic patient care products including supports, splints, restraints, braces, urinals, and other hospital supplies.

Ortho-Kinetics, Inc.
P.O. Box 436
Waukesha, Wisconsin 53187
1-800-558-12151

> Ortho-Kinetics carries a complete line of travel wheelchairs. Recently, Ortho-Kinetics introduced in the United States three products manufactured in Sweden: the Martin, probably the smallest wheelchair in the world; and the Minimax and Max, special chairs that offer a parent something between an umbrella stroller and a Travel Chair for a handicapped child.

Phonic Ear Ltd.
3060 Kerner Blvd.
San Rafael, California 94901
(415) 383-4000
> Phonic Ear Ltd. manufactures a full line of auditory training products for hearing impaired persons.

T.J. Posy Company
39 South Altadena Drive
Pasadena, California 91107
(213) 443-3143
> T.J. Posy Company carries a full line of patient safety aides such as vests, belts, restraints, and slings.

J.A. Preston Corporation
71 Fifth Avenue
New York, New York 10003
800-631-7277
> Preston Corporation offers materials for exceptional children through their Special Education Catalog. Their products include communication devices, therapeutic sensorimotor equipment and furniture.

Safety Travel Chairs, Inc.
147 Eady Court
Alyria, Ohio 44035
(216) 365-7593
> Safety Travel Chairs, Inc., specializes in manufacturing the Tran-Sporter wheelchair shown in Chapter 7, Figure 7.8. Safety Travel Chairs also make an adjustable prone board.

Index